OSTEOPATHIC MEDICINE

A Reformation in Progress

OSTEOPATHIC MEDICINE

A Reformation in Progress

R. MICHAEL GALLAGHER, DO
Vice Dean, School of Osteopathic Medicine
University of Medicine and Dentistry of New Jersey
Stratford, New Jersey

FREDERICK J. HUMPHREY, II, DO
Dean, School of Osteopathic Medicine
University of Medicine and Dentistry of New Jersey
Stratford, New Jersey

Consulting Editor **MARC S. MICOZZI**, MD, PhD

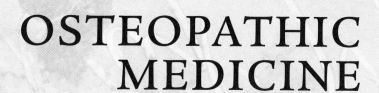

CHURCHILL LIVINGSTONE

A Harcourt Health Sciences Company
New York   Edinburgh   London   Philadelphia

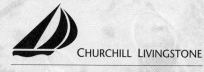

APR 2 0 2001

CHURCHILL LIVINGSTONE
A Harcourt Health Sciences Company

The Curtis Center
Independence Square West
Philadelphia, Pennsylvania 19106

Editor-in-Chief: John A. Schrefer
Editor: Kellie F. White
Associate Developmental Editor: Jennifer L. Watrous
Editorial Assistant: Becky Fuhrman
Project Manager: Gayle May Morris
Designer: Renée Duenow

OSTEOPATHIC MEDICINE   ISBN 0–443–07991–9

Printed in the United States of America.

Last digit is print number: 9   8   7   6   5   4   3   2   1

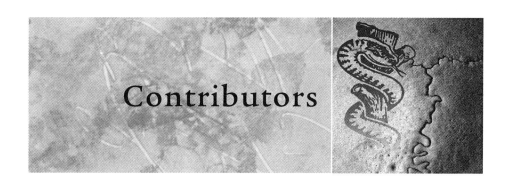

Contributors

R. MICHAEL GALLAGHER, DO
Vice Dean, Professor
School of Osteopathic Medicine
University of Medicine and Dentistry of New
   Jersey
Stratford, New Jersey

FREDERICK J. HUMPHREY, II, DO
Dean, Professor
School of Osteopathic Medicine
University of Medicine and Dentistry of New
   Jersey
Stratford, New Jersey

JOHN M. JONES, III, DO
Professor, Osteopathic Manipulative Medicine
Assistant Dean for Strategic Initiatives
Kirksville College of Osteopathic Medicine
Kirksville, Missouri

GERALD G. OSBORN, DO, M. Phil.
Professor of Psychiatry and Medicine
Adjunct Professor of History
College of Osteopathic Medicine
Michigan State University
East Lansing, Michigan

FELIX J. ROGERS, DO
Downriver Cardiology Consultants, P.C.
Trenton, Michigan

BARBARA ROSS-LEE, DO
Dean, Professor of Family Medicine
College of Osteopathic Medicine
Ohio University
Athens, Ohio

DOUGLAS L. WOOD, DO, PhD
President
American Association of Colleges of Osteopathic
   Medicine
Chevy Chase, Maryland

About the Authors

R. MICHAEL GALLAGHER, DO

R. Michael Gallagher, DO, FACOFP is Vice Dean and Professor of Family Medicine at the University of Medicine and Dentistry of New Jersey-School of Osteopathic Medicine in Stratford, New Jersey and serves on the Board of Governors of the American Association of Colleges of Osteopathic Medicine. He is an acknowledged leader in osteopathic medical education, particularly in primary care having served as Dean for Primary Care as well as Family Medicine Department Chair and Residency Program Director. He is Vice Chair of Council on Postdoctoral Training of the American Osteopathic Association and has served on the Council of Deans of the American Association of Colleges of Medicine. Dr. Gallagher's medical expertise is in the field of headache management and he is recognized internationally for his research and numerous publications. He is Board Certified in Family Medicine and Pain Management and is a Fellow of American College of Osteopathic Family Physicians, American Headache Society, College of Physicians of Philadelphia, and the Alliance of Air National Guard Flight Surgeons.

FREDERICK J. HUMPHREY, II, DO

Frederick J. Humphrey, II, DO, is Dean and Professor of Psychiatry at the University of Medicine and Dentistry of New Jersey-School of Osteopathic Medicine in Stratford, New Jersey. A leader in osteopathic medical education, Dr. Humphrey is currently Vice Chair of the OPTI (Osteopathic Postdoctoral Training Institution) Evaluation and Oversight Committee of the American Osteopathic Association. He has served as Chair of the Board of Governors of the American Association of Colleges of Osteopathic Medicine and Chair of the AOA Bureau of Professional Education. He is a graduate of the Institute of the Philadelphia Association of Psychoanalysis, is Board Certified in Adult and Child Psychiatry and is widely published in child psychiatry. Dr. Humphrey was formerly Associate Professor and Division Chief of Child Psychiatry and Vice-Chairman of the Department of Psychiatry at Penn State University College of Medicine-Milton S. Hershey Medical Center.

To Tracey Ellen and Robert Michael, II

R. MICHAEL GALLAGHER

To Babs, Fritz, Ian and Jessie
Thanks for all your support

FREDERICK J. HUMPHREY, II

Acknowledgements

Special thanks to Kathy Konicki, Jeff Bramnick, and Lawrence DeVaro

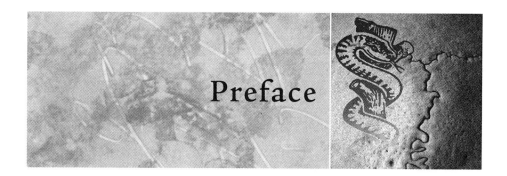

Preface

We've come a long way since A.T. Still set out to reform the practice of medicine a little more than a century ago. And the road has not been an easy one. It has been marked by countless obstacles, many still vivid and painful to recall.

Yet progress is clear. Osteopathic physicians fought for that progress, through years of scorn and derision, through years of labeling by allopathic physicians and some others, and through years of exclusion.

As osteopathic physicians, we answered the call for primary care long before it was popular to do so. The generalist-to-specialist ratio of the osteopathic system is the converse of the distribution within the allopathic system. Years of emphasis on structure and function have paid off in quality inpatient care and popularity among the general population of patients. And the years of hard work have paid us back with the establishment of our own identity. We've earned the respect of allopathic physicians and institutions, and we've earned the respect of the public, many of whom seek us out for their personal care.

Not too long ago, the major focus of osteopathic medicine: preventive care, manipulative medicine, communication with the patient, and a holistic approach, were viewed as radical and antiestablishment. But the winds of change have blown favorably for the osteopathic profession, bringing these once scorned ideals into vogue in the allopathic system. We have the opportunity now to be the leaders in meeting societal needs as medicine is transitioning from hospital-based care to ambulatory care.

Today osteopathic physicians practice in almost every conceivable environment and circumstance, in both osteopathic and traditionally allopathic institutions and settings. The numbers tell the story. Our numbers are growing: 30 years ago there were 5 osteopathic schools in the United States; today, there are 19, including 3 new schools in the last few years. And it doesn't stop there, as many older osteopathic institutions are expanding. In 1989 there were 25,000 osteopathic physicians in the United States. By the turn of the century the American Osteopathic Association reported 44,000 DOs in practice.

Sure, there are similarities between allopathic physicians and osteopathic physicians. Both want to further medicine and both strive for exemplary patient care. In 1999 the AAMC issued its report on the Medical School Objectives Project. One revealing section in the objectives states that students must have a "knowledge of the normal structure and function of the body (as an intact organism) and each of its major organ systems" and ". . . of the molecular, biochemical, and cellular mechanisms that are important in maintaining the body's homeostasis." Has a familiar ring, doesn't it?*

But, also there are differences. Our outlook is different. Our emphasis on structure and function and our hands-on approach make us distinct and set us apart. Our use of osteopathic manipulative therapy has enjoyed great success in treating myriad physical ailments and now draws interest from many allopathic physicians who want to learn the osteopathic manipulative medicine (OMM) techniques. There is much to be said for and about hands-on therapy. Our training, allowing students far greater clinical experience in ambulatory settings earlier in their medical education, prepares the osteopathic physicans of tomorrow with the skills they will need to build upon.

It's important that osteopathic physicians work together with those of the allopathic profession. But it's also important that we maintain our own identity in the community and beyond. Should we be cross-training with allopathic physicians? If so, how much is too much? Will this lead to greater blurring of the identity of our osteopathic hospitals and institutions? Will we simply melt into allopathic medicine?

These are weighty questions, to be sure. Remember, Dr. Still carved for us an identity. It is an identity that has continued to evolve. But if osteopathic medicine is to continue to have its own philosophy, its own identity, these are questions that every osteopathic physician must ask—and begin to answer.

This book is about where we've been, where we are, and where we're going. Of course, the purpose here is to inform. But there's more. The higher purpose of this book is to stimulate thought and meaningful discussion among those who care most about osteopathic medicine. It should serve as the light by which you arrive at your own thoughts about identity and our future.

Each of us should strive to leave osteopathic medicine a little better than we found it.

R. MICHAEL GALLAGHER
FREDERICK J. HUMPHREY, II

"Learning Objectives for Medical Student Education—Guidelines for Medical Schools: Report I of the Medical School Objectives Project," *Academic Medicine*, 74:1, 13-18.

An Open Letter to Osteopathic Students and Physicians

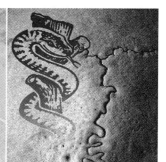

Osteopathic Medicine is at a crossroads. On all fronts we have made tremendous strides. On the political front, virtually all barriers have been overcome, creating our greatest challenge—yet the process of assimilating us has already begun. The majority of our graduates move directly into American College of Graduate Medical Education (ACGME) programs. Our hospitals have become generic and our graduates can be found on the faculties of the most prestigious allopathic medical schools. Allopathic medicine argues that there are no meaningful differences between us and welcomes our members into their country, state, and national medical societies and associations. Where do we go from here?! First we need to answer a number of key questions: Have we completed the reform movement that Andrew Taylor Still began so long ago? Have we accomplished on all fronts what we set out to do? Will our place in medical history be what we want it to be? Was the fight all of these years just for political equality or for something more?

In Chapter 6, "The Future," we have tried to stimulate debate by pointing out options. Everyone in the profession needs to arrive at their own conclusions, and then each of us needs to face the implications of those conclusions. These questions must be answered quickly since the assimilation process is well underway. It is all up to you! We can only shape our own destiny if *you* feel there are differences worth fighting for!

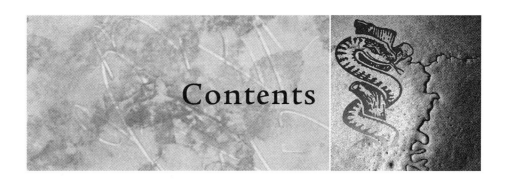

Contents

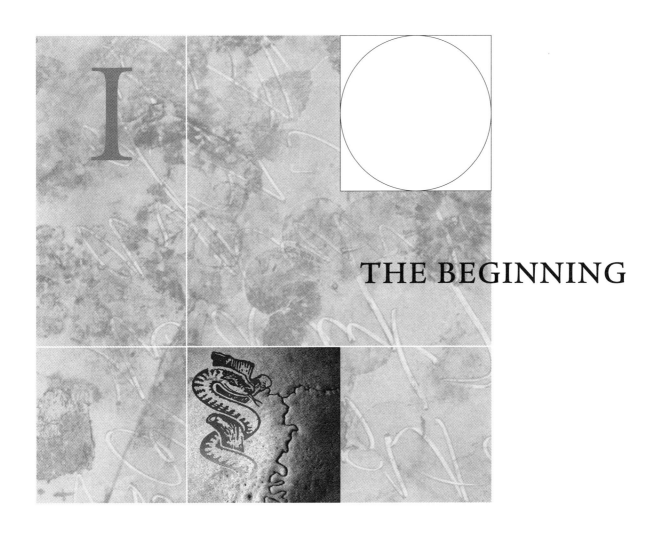

I

THE BEGINNING

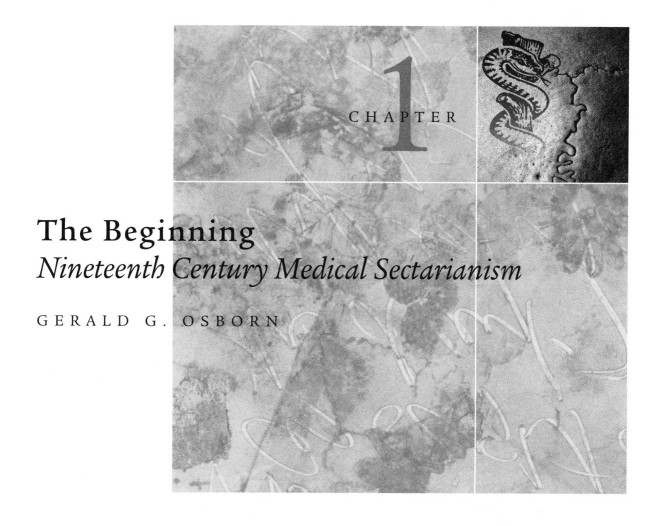

CHAPTER 1

The Beginning
Nineteenth Century Medical Sectarianism

GERALD G. OSBORN

*How much she bled, I have no means of judging, for I designedly prevented any
attempt to catch the blood and the convulsions were so violent and so frequent it
could not have been caught if attempted. I suffered her to bleed until the pulse could
not be felt at the wrist, and beat but feebly in the carotid arteries by which time the
convulsions ceased. . . .*

W.H. WHITT: "The Progress of Internal Medicine Since 1830," *The Centennial
History of the Tennessee Medical Association, 1830-1930,* Philip Hamer, ed., p. 265.

*A*merican medicine in the nineteenth century represented a collection
of highly variable groups of healers. America had a long tradition dating from its earliest colonial origins of lay domestic healing using
botanical preparations. This, combined in many places with botanic treatments
learned from Native American healers, formed the basis of most healing. At a level
above this fundamental health care were the physicians. They were a beleaguered
lot, struggling to make their individual livelihoods and form a true profession. In

terms of training and stature, American physicians were far removed from their counterparts in Western Europe. American educational institutions lagged far behind the developing scientific revolution sweeping Europe. This was most evident in medical education and training.

A unified pathway to becoming a physician did not exist in America in the nineteenth century. Medical schools did exist but varied widely in the quality of their education and training. They differed even on basic issues of requirements for entrance, curriculum, clinical opportunity, and length of study time needed to graduate. Apprenticeship was also a common parallel pathway to physicianhood. Many physicians with successful practices would take apprentices. After a period of usually 3 years of observing, studying, and assisting, the apprentice physician would be given a letter by his mentor attesting to his readiness to practice independently. Many physicians would choose a combination of both apprenticeship and medical school, providing them with both a degree and verification of their clinical experience.

Professional medical societies were in a fledgling developmental state as were state licensing and regulatory agencies. Many physicians, especially those in rural areas or in the territories, practiced solely on the basis of their apprentice letters or medical school diplomas. There were also elite American physicians from well-to-do families who attended medical school in Britain or on the Continent. Even those who trained at the older and more established American medical schools in the East would go to Europe for graduate specialty training, especially in surgery. All would eventually return to America to highly successful practices, usually in large cities.[4] These elite physicians composed a distinct and very powerful minority within the American medical establishment. Another point of division was the sectarian nature of American medical education and practice. Three major and distinct medical sects were well established by the mid nineteenth century, each with its own theories about the etiology of disease and its proper treatment. The three sects constantly argued, bickered, and at times even had physical confrontations with one another. These groups had different origins, different medical schools, and different ideas about therapeutics.

REGULARS OR ALLOPATHS

The regular physicians were by far the more numerous and well established of the sects. Although they had the most medical schools and hospitals, many continued to receive their training by apprenticeship only. These physicians were politically powerful; they formed local and state medical societies, with varying degrees of internal strife, dating back to the colonial period. When the New York State Medical Society tried to raise the standards of the medical schools in their state, they were met with resistance by the schools themselves. They reasoned that if New York raised the schools' standards, prospective medical students might be drawn to other institutions outside the state. To prevent this occurrence, formation of a national organization would be necessary if standards were to be raised.

A national convention was organized in 1846 in New York amidst an atmosphere of skepticism and mistrust. Many medical schools refused to attend, but nevertheless, it aroused interest sufficient that a second convention was held in Philadelphia the following year. The 1847 meeting was much better attended, and the founding of the American Medical Association (AMA) was the result. Far from abolishing apprenticeship as a pathway to becoming a physician, the convention participants declared certain standards should be met before a person could qualify as being an approved preceptor for future physicians. Of the 19 medical schools that responded to the American Medical Association's first survey, only 12 of them required any clinical instruction at all, and only 5 required dissection in their curriculum. The AMA and its affiliate societies also began to strongly lobby the state legislatures' regulatory boards to support them in their endeavors to set higher standards.[16]

Heroic Therapies

Even though the regulars represented the majority of physicians, academic historians of medicine agree their dogmatic postures regarding health, illness, and therapeutics easily qualify them as sectarian practitioners.[14] No unified system of diagnosis existed, and disease was felt to be the particular constellation of symptoms any ill person exhibited. The basis of most therapy consisted of blood-letting, purging (from above and below) and blistering. These treatments could be used singly or in any combination, based on the physicians' judgements in any clinical circumstance. These active and dramatically interventive therapeutics date back to classical antiquity and were vigorously defended by even the most elegantly educated elite.

Bleeding of the patients was performed by a number of methods, the most common being a longitudinal cut of a vein (occasionally an artery) with a scalpel or lancet. Purging was most commonly accomplished by administering a chalky mercury preparation called "Calomel." Mercury is a toxic irritant to mucous membranes and the lining of the gastrointestinal tract and causes profuse salivation, violent vomiting, and diarrhea. Physicians would determine the dose of Calomel by the severity of the inflammation on the patients' lips, gums, and oral mucous membranes. The purpose was to cleanse the stomach and bowels of impurities that might be causing or contributing to the illness. Finally, blistering was achieved by many methods ranging from the use of heated metal to more benign mildly irritating plasters. This technique was usually performed on a part of the body opposite of where the illness was thought to be located. If the illness was deemed systemic, the blistering could be either multiple or singular on a broad body surface. Blistering was thought to draw the toxins from the illness to the body surface, which would then be drained away. Regular physicians believed these techniques served to actively remove toxic substances from the sick person.

These practices were the mainstay of regular therapeutics and were taught in medical schools and apprenticeships alike well into the early twentieth century. This tenacity is represented in some of the later writings of Sir William Osler of Johns Hopkins, arguably the most famous regular physician of the time. His 1912 journal article discusses blood-letting in the treatment of respiratory disease. "To bleed at the outset in pneumonia in robust and healthy individuals in whom the disease sets-in with great intensity and high fever is, I believe, a good practice and small amounts are often insufficient."[14] In Osler's *Textbook of Medicine,* he recommends, "a dose of Calomel during the day to open the bowels," as a component of the treatment for influenza.[11] Osler continued to use Calomel his entire medical career, and it continued to be used as a staple medication by regular physicians as late as 1937.[14]

The obvious unpleasant nature of these therapies makes it difficult to comprehend why adults would submit to them, let alone allow their children to receive them also. The answers lie in the supreme confidence of most physicians using them, the trust, and in many cases the desperation of the patients, and finally, the paucity of other professionally valid therapeutic alternatives. Again medical historians argue quite persuasively that until the second half of the nineteenth century only three valid therapies existed, cinchona bark for aches and fever, inoculation and vaccination for small pox, and direct surgical interventions for infection and gangrene; in most cases this meant amputation.[14] The "valid" therapies combined with the heroic "invalid" therapies were the primary treatment armamentarium of the regulars.

Not all of the regulars were completely sanguine about medical heroics. Dr. J. Marion Simms wrote shortly after medical school graduation in 1835 that "the practice of medicine of the time is heroic: it was murderous. I knew nothing about medicine but still had sense enough to see that doctors were killing their patients."[14] Simms was not alone, but in a distinct minority. Even among those physicians increasingly skeptical of heroic treatment, few would step forward to criticize it openly. Jacob Bigelow, another prominent regular, wrote, "so great at one time was . . . the ascending of heroic teachers and writers, that few medical men had the courage to incur the responsibility of omitting the active modes of treatment which were deemed indispensable."[14] For Bigelow, Simms, and others, any reasonable alternatives were bound to have tremendous appeal. These alternatives would also be welcomed by their patients.

HOMEOPATHY

Law of Similars

The first major challenge to heroic therapies came from an increasingly skeptical regular physician, formally educated and trained in Germany. Samuel Christian Friedreich Hahnemann (Figure 1-1) became so disillusioned with heroic therapies that he ceased to practice for a time and looked for answers within classical texts that he was translating into German. In 1790 while testing on himself the potency of a solution of cinchona bark, he noticed that it produced in him the same effects as malaria, the disease it was supposed to cure. Informed by his extensive knowledge of ancient texts and biblical references about the causes and treatment of illness, he now had a revelation following this personal and pivotal experience.[6] He hypothesized that agents that caused the symptoms of any illness in a healthy person were the cure for the same illness in a sick person. He called his revolutionary new theory "similia, similibus curantur": "likes cure," or "the law of similars."

He further elaborated his new method to include systematic testing for all medications. He called these new tests "provings." They consisted of healthy subjects taking various medicines and carefully recording the symptoms they experienced. These provings were used to match medications with the same symp-

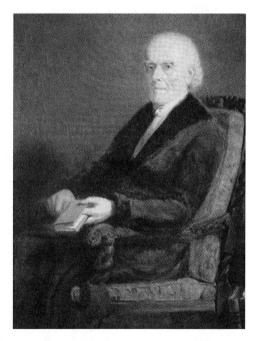

Figure 1-1 Dr. Samuel Hahnemann (1755-1843) founded homeopathy on the premise that drugs producing certain symptoms in healthy people will cure those same symptoms in the sick. (From Richardson S: *Homeopathy: Stimulating the Body's Natural Immune System,* Harmony Books, New York, 1988.)

toms seen in a person who is ill. Hahnemann also hypothesized that the process of diluting these medications actually increased their efficacy and further that vigorously shaking the dilute mixture (dynamization) immediately before taking it increased its efficacy even more. He placed great emphasis on spending sufficient time with each patient to take a detailed history of the evolution of symptoms over time. He also placed extreme importance on the purity of medications and precision in their preparation (Figure 1-2). He supported his theory of the efficacy of minute doses by comparing it to the efficacy of inoculation and vaccination to prevent small pox. Later he proposed a generic theory of the etiology of all disease being a suppressed itch or "psora." It was this last theory that caused him to be ridiculed by regular practitioners and other sectarians.[14] Hahnemann called his new medical system *homeopathy*. He also coined the term *allopathy* for the system of diagnosis and treatment provided by regular physicians: a name many resented bitterly.

From the unempathetic and even hostile perspective of the allopaths, Hahnemann's therapeutics appeared to be merely offering a small drink of water to sick patients. Patients, however, experienced being treated by a well-trained, caring physician who spent much more time with them and provided a treatment that neither hurt nor incapacitated them for days. Homeopathic treatment was at least as efficacious as allopathic care and, given the harm caused by heroic therapies, was probably far superior. Hahnemann's formal German medical education and early academic posts at the university medical schools of Leipsic and Dresden provided him with the legitimacy needed to begin to teach his system to other physicians. The care and precision of his methods and their wide anecdotal efficacy compared to heroic therapies provided other disillusioned regulars a reasonable alternative. At least homeopathic treatment was consistent with the Hippocratic

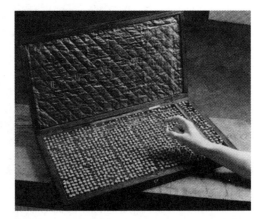

Figure 1-2 Samuel Hahnemann's remedy box. Many homeopaths kept their remedies in a similar box, but few had one that was so splendid. (From Richardson S: *Homeopathy: Stimulating the Body's Natural Immune System,* Harmony Books, New York, 1988.)

aphorism "Primum Non Nocere, First do no harm." Homeopathy spread across Western Europe, becoming very popular with the upper classes. Hahnemann died in Paris a successful and very wealthy man.[7]

Homeopathy in America

Homeopathy came to America by two separate and independent routes. Hans Gram was an American who studied medicine in Europe and was persuaded by Hahnemann's ideas. He returned in 1825 to New York City, developed a successful upper class practice, and began to teach others this new system. He began by using the common alternative pathway of educating by taking on apprentices and training them in Hahnemann's methods. He was almost singularly responsible for homeopathy's early foothold in New York City. The second and more important wave of homeopaths were those trained in Europe who then immigrated to America. The most prominent of these was Constantine Hering, who founded the first homeopathic medical school in Allentown, Pennsylvania in 1833, its instruction given entirely in German. In 1841 he obtained a charter for the Homeopathic Medical College of Pennsylvania in Philadelphia with its instruction in English. This second medical school flourished and made Philadelphia the national center of training in homeopathy.[5] With homeopathy's appeal to regular physicians skeptical of heroic therapies, the ranks of converts began to grow and spread west across America. By the end of the nineteenth century there were homeopathic medical schools in many large American cities including Philadelphia, New York City, Boston, Chicago, and even Ann Arbor, Michigan and Iowa City, Iowa.

Controversies arose within the American homeopathic ranks. On the conservative side were the Hahnemannian *high dilutionists* who fought to preserve original teachings and methods. The liberal side consisted of many former allopaths who were persuaded by some of Hahnemann's ideas but who found many of his teachings and ideas difficult to accept, such as dynamization, high dilutions, and all illness resulting from the suppressed itch. These *low dilutionist practitioners* became more numerous and eventually were able to be coopted and merged into the larger American allopathic system. This did not happen, however, until American homeopathy had created its own extensive network of societies, medical schools, hospitals, journals, and even separate state licensing boards. Their education and training was recognized to be at least equal to many of the leading allopathic schools, with the major difference being the teaching of the homeopathic system of therapeutics. A number of prominent medical schools today had their origins in the homeopathic sect— MCP–Hahnemann University, now part of Allegeheny University; New York Medical College; Boston University; University of Iowa; and University of Michigan, to name a few.

MEDICAL ECLECTICISM

America had a long tradition of botanical healing dating back to its earliest colonial times. This tradition became increasingly elaborate and developed into lay apprenticeships and later even into "Friendly Societies" of botanical healing. This process was aided by the publication of a number of books and manuals for use within the home; the most famous of these being *A New Guide to Health* by Samuel Thomson. Thomson was a farmer who disliked farming as much as he did the pretensions of regular physicians and their heroic practices. He marketed his manual of botanic therapy through a system of societies, becoming very successful and wealthy in the process.[14] As Thomson's and others' methods became increasingly elaborate, it was only a matter of time before this movement became professionalized.

The first group derived directly from the Thomsonian movement was led by Alva Curtis, a professional botanic healer. He and his supporters were able to establish a number of botanical medical schools. Another group was led by Wooster Beach who was a formally trained allopath who then apprenticed with a botanical healer. In 1830 he and other regular physicians disillusioned with heroic practices established a medical school in Worthington, Ohio. Their medical school was successful until a scandal involving a missing corpse caused a riot in town leading to the closure of the school in 1840. Faculty from the school, and later Beach himself, developed a new medical school in Cincinnati, Ohio that became the center of training for professional botanical medicine—the Eclectic Medical Institute of Cincinnati.

These botanical practitioners called themselves *medical eclectics* because they were against most, but not all, of the heroic therapies and open to novel treatment modalities as they developed. They strongly rejected bleeding and blistering but retained purging as an effective treatment. Their purging was, of course, with the use of botanical preparations and never with a harsh inorganic substance like Calomel. These new sectarians were harshly received by allopaths and homeopaths alike. They therefore continued to develop, as did the homeopaths, their own medical schools, societies, infirmaries, and medical journals. The medical eclectics were never able to gain equal stature with the other sectarians. At their peak they had only 10 medical schools, and only three or four of these were reasonably funded and provided a training course comparable to the other sects. Their medical school in Cincinnati was by far the most successful and continued as an independent institution until 1939. The eclectics were most successful in the rural Midwest, and their patients were generally from the working and lower classes.[15]

OSTEOPATHY

The three original medical sects in America were joined by a late-comer in 1874. As with the homeopaths and eclectics, it was a reform movement against heroic therapeutics. It was, however, neither a European import nor a professionalized lay movement, but came instead from within the ranks of orthodox American regular medical practice.

Founder of Osteopathy

Andrew Taylor Still (1828-1917) was the son of a Methodist minister and medical missionary. His early formal education was better than most. His medical training was for all intents and purposes completely orthodox and consistent with the pathway of apprenticeship, mostly under his father's instruction. He supplemented his knowledge by studying medical texts and dissected bodies from an Indian burial ground to increase his understanding of anatomy. He received additional training and experience during the Civil War, first as an enlisted man serving as a hospital steward and later as a commissioned officer, reaching the rank of Major in the 21st Kansas Militia.

Following military service he returned to orthodox medical practice, but his faith in regular medicine was soon to be shaken forever. The pivotal time came in the spring of 1864 when his family became ill with meningitis. His orthodoxy is clearly demonstrated by his summoning of his physician colleagues to treat his family. Still watched as the heroic therapies of his colleagues failed and in the end three of his family lay dead. The experience lead him in the direction of therapeutic skepticism but, initially, without an alternative.[17] Historians of osteopathy point to an amalgam of developmental experiences that inspired Still to move away from orthodoxy after the death of his family.[3] These include the temperate belief system of Methodism and some early exposure to "drugless" therapies including magnetic healing.

Temperance in all things was consistent with the popular health movement of Sylvester Graham. Graham's *Lectures on the Science of Human Life* outlined general principles of moderation that, if people followed, would result in them getting sick less often and, if they did get ill, would enhance their bodies' natural recuperative powers and would shorten their recovery time. However, it was a combination of ideas from magnetic healing and the very practical craft of bone-setting from which Still derived his inspiration. Magnetic healing combined spiritualism and healing by seeking to restore the balance of an invisible magnetic fluid circulating throughout the body. The balance was restored by massage and verbal suggestion as well as proper placement of the body within an external magnetic field. Still did not accept the entire spiritual dimension of the magnetic therapy but was persuaded by the metaphor of the harmonious balance of the interaction of body parts and the unobstructed flow of body fluids. He embraced the therapeutic technique to the point that he advertised himself as a "magnetic healer" when he opened a practice in Kirksville, Missouri in 1874.

Bone-setting was a craft that was brought to early colonial America by European immigrants. Bone-setting began as an apprenticed-trained craft that dealt only with the reduction of fractures and dislocations. As the craft became more elaborate, it expanded to include manipulation of any joint thought to be diseased or even minimally "out of place." Many patients with joints restricted by arthritis or long-standing prior injury were helped by bonesetters trained in this expanded fashion (Figure 1-3).

How Still received his training in bone-setting remains obscure, but it was probably obtained by observing a practitioner in an apprentice-style manner. Any new skill would have been to Still's economic benefit as it would greatly expand his patient population. Sometime in the 1880s he began to advertise himself as a "lightening bone-setter."[13] When he used some manipulative techniques to treat the thoracic spine and ribs of a woman with asthma with good results, he reported, "it started me on a new train of thought."[3] Also obscure in Still's background is the source of his association with some engineering principles.[20] The first rule of engineering, "form follows function," inspired his novel and unified doctrine of health, illness, and treatment.

Once informed by a constellation of developmental beliefs and experiences, he hypothesized that the concept of magnetic healing was correct. However, rather than universal magnetic fluid being obstructed, he thought it was actually the obstruction of the flow of blood and lymph. The obstruction was caused by some

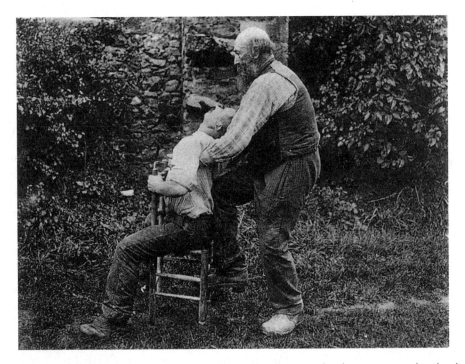

Figure 1-3 This French postcard shows a bonesetter treating a lumbago or acute low back pain. It was shot in Britanny, France, near Vannes, circa 1880. (Courtesy Musee des Arts et Traditions Populaires, Paris, France.)

compromise in the skeletal structure of the patient, the result of either injury or illness. His simple concept of structure being reciprocally related to function became his central diagnostic and therapeutic tenet: Disease is caused or promoted by some compromise in the structural integrity of the body and can be reflected by careful examination of the musculoskeletal system. This compromised integrity obstructs the flow of bodily fluids, especially blood, and the resulting imbalance gives rise to specific symptoms of disease. Still's abandoned heroic therapies could now be positively replaced by this new method, in which the body would be systematically examined, diagnosed, and restored to proper function by restoring proper structure.

Still began medical practice anew, using his new system of healing to treat all illness. This new method of treatment was clearly never meant to treat only musculoskeletal disorders but as a comprehensive new approach to the diagnosis and treatment of illness in general. Still made an attempt to present his novel ideas at Baker University in Baldwin, Kansas but was turned away. His physician colleagues likewise criticized him harshly or at the very least distanced themselves from him. Still then took his family to Missouri, first to Macon but shortly thereafter to Kirksville.

His new practice in Kirksville was too small to sustain a reasonable life for his family, and he was forced to become an itinerant physician serving a number of surrounding communities. His income began to improve, but his reputation continued to be quite mixed. Gradually, testimonials about the efficacy of his care began to spread, and people began to anxiously anticipate his arrival in their community. His practice in Kirksville did not flourish, however, until he successfully treated the daughter of the local Presbyterian minister. The minister, Rev. J. K. Mitchell had prior to this event shunned Still's methods and ideas, but Mrs. Mitchell surreptitiously took their daughter to receive this novel therapy while her husband was away. For some time this young girl had been unable to walk. After a series of manipulative treatments she was able to walk down the stairs to greet her father on his return home. The minister then became not only a believer but a proponent of Still. Still's practice grew in respectability and, most importantly, in income allowing him to practice exclusively in Kirksville.

Still received national attention when he treated the son of United States Senator Foraker of Missouri. Foraker's son had "valvular disease of the heart" and regular physicians gave the family no hope for the boy's survival. After treatment by Still, the boy improved and survived into middle age, and Senator Foraker became a life-long advocate of this new therapy.[21] Still's reputation spread to the point of being able to establish his own infirmary by 1889, and patients traveled from great distances seeking this new form of treatment. The dramatic success led Still to both name his discovery and establish a school to teach and train others. Since he was using primarily the skeletal system as levers to perform his style of manipulation, he felt the Greek root *os* (osteon) was aptly descriptive. Since other forms of healing used "pathy," that is, allopathy and homeopathy, (derived from *pathos,* Greek for suffering), he entitled his discovery "osteopathy" and opened his American School of Osteopathy in 1892.

Humble Origins of Osteopathy

It is most important here to provide the professional context in which this most recent sectarian movement was to begin its struggle. Still's American School of Osteopathy (ASO) was started in a small house that he purchased with his personal savings (Figure 1-4). Almost simultaneously in Baltimore, Maryland, with $7 million of donated money, Johns Hopkins University opened its medical school in 1893. This striking contrast in resources takes the term *uneven playing field* to almost absurd levels.[16]

The ASO's future was given its early opportunity for success by the chance visit to Kirksville of Dr. William Smith, a Scottish surgeon. Smith was trained at the medical school of the University of Edinburgh, arguably one of the finest in the world. He was in America looking for expanded markets for British-made surgical instruments. He heard of Still's plan for a new medical school and, seeing this as a prospect for business, met with Still and was astonished but also intrigued by their discussions. Smith's initial skepticism was overcome by his sense that Still's ideas and new endeavor had merit, and he agreed to stay and teach

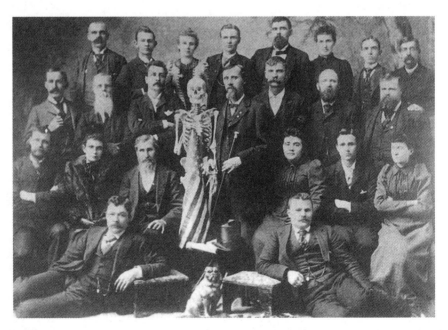

Figure 1-4 A. T. Still's first class (1892) at the American School of Osteopathy in Kirksville, Missouri. (Courtesy Still National Museum of Osteopathy, Kirksville, Missouri.)

both anatomy and surgery at the school. The school became so well known that the number of patients seen in its infirmary increased to the point where more trains had to be scheduled to Kirksville to transport all the people seeking treatment. In addition to William Smith, Still was ultimately able to attract a well-qualified faculty, many of whom eventually left to establish osteopathic schools elsewhere. Amongst these were the Littlejohn brothers, also from Britain. James and David were physicians trained in Glasgow, Scotland and Michigan respectively. J. Martin Littlejohn had both law and divinity degrees from Glasgow and a PhD in political science from Columbia in New York. Each of the brothers had prior positive experiences with osteopathy and came to Kirksville anxious to teach and to learn.

Although he was a skillful innovator and seasoned clinician, Still was hardly a scholar. His descriptions of his method were convoluted, and his teaching methods primarily made use of analogy and parable. The faculty he gathered, however, were able to assist him with articulating his methods more clearly and helped shape the further elaboration of osteopathy. The faculty were also able to connect the basic concepts of osteopathy with other emerging medical theories. Ultimately, ASO's faculty provided the academic and intellectual legitimacy necessary for the profession to survive.

For a short time an internal struggle developed between those early doctors of osteopathy (DOs) who wished osteopathy to remain purely a manipulative method of healing and those who wished it to develop a more comprehensive approach and yet keep the structure-function paradigm central. The debate became known as the "lesionists" versus the "broads." Still would have ranked somewhere in the middle-ground of this debate, upset with the lesionists for being so narrow but also suspicious of the broads for seeming too quick to incorporate new ideas and methods. The broads won Still over, and eventually the ASO's curriculum expanded and the length of study increased to that of many allopathic medical colleges.

Osteopathy's successes did not go unnoticed by the other sectarian groups. Each of the other three groups in Missouri stopped bickering amongst themselves long enough to cooperatively introduce a bill to the House of Representatives in 1893 that would require practitioners of osteopathy to also be graduates of a "reputable" medical school. It was too little too late. Lawmakers were deluged by letters and telegrams from osteopathy's supporters and the bill failed. However, osteopathic graduates were not allowed to join medical societies, admit patients to other sectarian hospitals, or participate in their specialty training programs. Just as the other sects had done, osteopathy had to develop its own organizations, hospitals, and schools, and did so as expeditiously as possible. The new movement saw the need for a national organization, and in 1897 the American Association for the Advancement of Osteopathy was founded. The next year the name was changed to the American Osteopathic Association (AOA). Soon after its creation, the AOA organized into divisional societies and began to strategically work toward nationwide professional recognition for its members.

Legal Recognition

Recognizing that securing legal recognition equivalent to that of the other sects was its most important task, the AOA formed a Committee on Legislation in 1901. The struggle for legal recognition from state to state ranged from easy and quick to strenuous political battles taking many years. Not surprisingly, Missouri was the first state to legally recognize osteopathy as being equivalent to the recognition of MD's (Doctor of Medicine) but not without strenuous opposition from the other sects.

Michigan was a different case entirely. State Representative Caroll, who was also the Postmaster in Grand Rapids, had been traveling to Chicago to receive osteopathic manipulative treatment. He disliked having to travel such distances to receive his treatments and hoped to recruit osteopathic physicians to Michigan. Simultaneously, State Senator Moore, after reading an article about the successful treatment of U.S. Senator Foraker's child by osteopathic treatment, introduced a bill to formally recognize osteopathy in Michigan. Together Caroll and Moore stewarded their legislation through both chambers of the legislature, and it was signed into law by then Governor H. S. Pingree on 21 April 1897.[1] This occurred prior to the state having any active osteopathic practitioners. This early and easily won legal recognition would have far-reaching implications not only for osteopathy's future survival but also for its ability to thrive.

State by state legal recognition was achieved by three general methods: (1) the creation of a distinct osteopathic board of examiners, (2) the formation of a composite board with osteopathic representation, and (3) a medical board that agreed to examine and license DOs. In California, as in Missouri, legal recognition was harshly opposed by MDs, but ultimately the DOs were sufficiently organized to win approval of the formation of a distinct board for instituting osteopathic examination and licensure in 1901. In stark contrast are the states of Louisiana and Mississippi where strong MD opposition prevented equivalent osteopathic licensure until 1973. Some states created two levels of osteopathic licensure, one exclusively for manipulative treatment and one for full-scope licensure as MDs enjoyed. Because the scope of training in osteopathic medical schools expanded, the use of these lower-level practice licenses gradually disappeared.

Survival and Gradual Growth

Almost identical to the progression of other sectarian schools, osteopathic medical schools began to proliferate with a wide range of academic quality. National associations representing each of the sects became increasingly concerned with raising the standards of their education and training. This meant raising premedical criteria for entrance, improving the quality of basic and clinical training, and increasing the length of study necessary to graduate.

The most expansive and best-funded examination of medical school proliferation was the Flexner Report. The American Medical Association in 1906 inspected the then 160 schools granting MD degrees and fully approved only 82. The AMA then invited the Carnegie Foundation for the Advancement of Teaching to conduct an even more comprehensive survey. On the recommendation of Dr. Simon Flexner, a Johns Hopkins graduate and then president of the Rockefeller Institute for Medical Research, his younger brother Abraham, a school teacher, was hired to carry out the inspections. Abraham also had received his bachelors degree from Johns Hopkins University.

Accompanied by the secretary of the AMA's Council on Medical Education, Abraham Flexner visited every medical school in America. Based on the preliminary correspondence he sent to each medical school, they believed him to be on a scouting mission for a major philanthropic organization. With hopes for grants and endowments, most medical school administrations anxiously anticipated Flexner's visit.

Such hopes were dashed when the outcome of the survey proved Abraham Flexner to be an elitist. In the famous "Bulletin Number Four," he affirmed that the highest requirements for a medical education were represented by the medical school of Johns Hopkins University. Flexner strongly recommended the closure of the vast majority of medical schools in America; only 31 of them received his approval. His critique of sectarian medical schools other than allopathic was especially harsh.[2]

Rather than crediting Flexner for the subsequent reform of medical schools, a number of medical historians now indicate that effective reform was well underway prior to Flexner, and at most, his "Bulletin Number Four" merely hastened the demise of the poorest medical schools and deprived them of their mourners. Flexner recognized that there was a gradual push for higher standards already underway and that economic considerations would be responsible for culling the financially strapped proprietary medical schools.[16] The AOA Committee on Education responded to the Flexner report by implementing their own process of slow, steady reform for those osteopathic medical colleges that survived the waves of closings and consolidations.

The osteopathic profession faced an enormous disadvantage during this time because they received no state or federal support, no tax support, and little assistance from philanthropic organizations. Because they also concentrated their efforts on producing generalist clinical practitioners, they received little in extramural funding to build a research base. Osteopathic medical schools also continued to provide a pathway for the disadvantaged, that is, the poor, women, and minorities, to become physicians. Although elitist Flexner was unsympathetic to these issues, the admissions committees of osteopathic medical schools stead-fastly continued to consider a wide spectrum of candidates.

Again for the sake of contrast, Johns Hopkins agreed to admit women to its medical school only after receiving a $500 thousand endowment created by do-nations from wealthy women. In regard to research, between the publication in 1910 of "Bulletin Number Four" and 1936, the Rockefeller Institute's General Ed-ucation Board provided $91 million to select allopathic medical schools, with seven of them receiving over two thirds of the total amount.[16]

 Even with this financial inequity, the quality of osteopathic medical schools began to improve during this time, but at a much slower pace than did the other medical institutions. Also, since DOs were being prevented from pursuing grad-uate medical education and training within MD institutions, they began to ex-pand their own system of hospitals. Many DOs early in the twentieth century, by a variety of means, still were able to acquire MD degrees that enabled them to get a broader spectrum of specialty training. Most continued to identify themselves with the osteopathic profession, and they became the vanguard for the expansion of osteopathic specialty training, especially in the areas of surgery and internal medicine.

When a significant number of DOs opened their practices within a geographic area, they would usually buy and refurbish a large old home and turn it into an in-firmary or small hospital. As osteopathic hospital boards became more sophisti-cated, they would negotiate financing, buy property, and then build a small hos-pital from the ground up. Gradual improvement in education standards resulted in the expansion of full licensure in an increasing number of states and some ex-ternal recognition. The College of Osteopathic Physicians and Surgeons in Los Angeles, for example, was able to acquire access to a county hospital for clinical training and patient care.

As time progressed, the sects of homeopathy and medical eclecticism were be-ing absorbed into the allopathic mainstream. However, the DOs continued to be confronted persistently with hostile campaigns organized against them by mem-bers of the allopathic medicine community that were designed to constrain the growth of and, ultimately, to eliminate the osteopathic profession altogether. But the severity of the uneven playing field was not to continue.

Thriving and Explosive Growth

As America entered World War II, many MDs were drafted into military service. DOs were not recognized as equivalent at that time by the armed forces and there-for could not serve as commissioned medical officers. DOs were, however, equiv-alently licensed in most states, and many of them received exemption from the draft to provide health care to the country. Many former patients of MDs then went to DOs and found the care of sufficiently high quality to continue going even after the end of the war. During the war allopathic hospitals continued their strict ban against granting admitting privileges to DOs, which resulted in a further expansion of osteopathic hospitals to accommodate the increased number of patients receiving care from DOs.

The AOA began the private Osteopathic Progress Fund during World War II, which netted $962,535, primarily from DOs and grateful patients, in its first campaign. These funds were distributed among the osteopathic colleges to be used for program improvement. Between 1946 and 1961 this fund effort raised $8,956,625 in private support for osteopathic education. In 1946 the Hill Burton Act recognized the osteopathic profession as being eligible for major grants for hospital construction. By 1956, the profession was also recognized by the U.S. Public Health Service as eligible for renewable teaching grants. Many returning veterans used the G.I. Bill to fund their education at osteopathic medical schools. This positive slant of the "playing field" toward osteopathic medicine increased standards even more, developed residency programs within the expanded hospital system, and further increased the number of states granting full licensure to DOs.

Osteopathic physicians had always scored significantly higher than foreign medical graduates on both basic science and clinical examinations as measured by the composite licensing boards. The higher standards of the schools were reflected by osteopathic physicians gradually achieving licensing examination scores approximating those of the American MDs graduating from much better funded institutions. Ironically, even using data from as far back as the early 1940s showing that American osteopathic physicians scored much higher on the same medical licensing examinations than did foreign-trained physicians, foreigners who passed the medical examinations were eligible for allopathic specialty training, but DOs were continually denied.[3]

Merger in California

The new and fairly rapid upward movement of the profession did not come early enough for many DOs who were unhappy with their position relative to that of MDs. California was seen by many as the flagship osteopathic state with the most practitioners, the largest medical school, and the largest number of hospitals. Even with these advantages, DOs suffered from "status inconsistency," that is, they had training equivalent to their MD counterparts but continued to suffer discrimination at every turn. Also, as the curriculum expanded for all osteopathic colleges, training in osteopathic manipulation began to take a more peripheral role.

Graduates from the California school, especially, felt this had happened to such a degree that there were so many more commonalities than differences in the education of DOs and MDs that there was little reason to stay separate. As early as 1943 discussions about a merger had occurred between the California Osteopathic and California Medical Associations. By this time homeopathy and medical eclecticism had been fully assimilated into the mainstream medical community, and many felt it was time for osteopathy to take that path as well. After a number of abortive attempts, the California Osteopathic Association (COA) and the California Medical Association (CMA) achieved closure on a merger agreement in 1961. The agreement provided that the osteopathic college would change its name to the California College of Medicine and would now award the MD degree. The offer of an MD degree from this institution would be extended to all living graduates as well as any DO in California who held a full license to practice. All DOs who accepted the MD degree had to cease identifying themselves as osteopathic physicians, and the California College of Medicine would cease to teach osteopathic principles and practice.

The agreement on future licensing, however, became the most onerous and hotly contested issue of the merger. The COA agreed to support legislation that would prevent any new DOs from being licensed in the state. The separate osteopathic licensing board would retain jurisdiction over those DOs in the state who refused the MD degree. When those DO practitioners dwindled to under 40 in number, the board would be forever abolished. After the window to accept the MD degree closed, DOs would be permanently restricted from practicing in California.[16]

Amidst an atmosphere of jubilation, over 2000 DOs paid $65 for their new MD degrees in a large auditorium in Los Angeles County General Hospital on the 14th and 15th of July 1961. "We thought we had won the war. Many of us went to merger parties afterwards and celebrated the victory. Absolutely no more being discriminated against or having to explain what an osteopath is."[9] These statements by former DOs turned out to be only partially correct. For each former DO, the issue of explaining their degree to people unknowledgeable about the profession did indeed instantaneously disappear. The discrimination, however, did not end.

The new DOs were accepted into the CMA but were segregated for a long period into a separate forty-first society. Their MD was an "academic" rather than a "professional" degree, recognized only within the state of California. Those former DOs who were specialists certified by their respective osteopathic specialty boards quickly discovered continued discrimination if they moved and presented their specialty qualifications to allopathic hospitals. If they moved to an institution that was a former osteopathic hospital they were generally still well received. Former DO specialists who remained in their established practices were generally not affected by the loss of their board certification. Board certification did not have the same critical importance for hospital staff privileges as it does today, and many specialists managed quite well never sitting for specialty examinations after their residency programs.

The winners in the California merger seemed to be those former DO general practitioners and former DO specialists for whom board certification credentials were not critical to their future. General practitioners at that time had neither residency programs nor specialty boards. Most generalists, both MD and DO, went into practice immediately after completing their internships.

Another big winner was the University of California system. The former private College of Osteopathic Physicians and Surgeons, now the California College of Medicine, became incorporated into a state school at the University of California, Irvine where it remains today. The major winner, however, was the allopathic profession, which acquired over 2000 new members, many new hospitals, and a new medical school without much expenditure of either money or political concessions. The loser at first pass seemed to be the osteopathic profession as a whole, which was now being barred from practicing in California, one of the most popular states in which to practice medicine.

Many within and outside the osteopathic profession felt the merger in California to be the first major step on the path already taken by homeopathy and medical eclecticism and fully expected a wave of state-by-state mergers in the near future. It was not to happen. Merger attempts were made by other DOs disgruntled by their lack of allopathic acceptance and impatient with the pace of progress the profession was making toward equality. Most merger negotiations were unsuccessful because they lacked the numbers of practitioners and level of organization the DOs had in California. Also, allopathic feelings about DOs elsewhere were much more strongly negative, and many merger offers were met with scorn. In the state of Washington a group of DOs even negotiated a merger with the state medical society and founded a bogus medical school, the Washington College of Physicians and Surgeons offering an MD degree. The Washington State Board of Medical Examiners agreed to accept the degree for licensing. Litigation by DOs against the merger was successful in exposing the sham and closing the "medical school" but not until the affair reached the State Supreme Court.[3] Organized osteopathic medicine was successful in holding the profession together, but many DOs felt their future was still uncertain.

Merger Aftermath

The facts of the California merger became widely known and became very politically useful to the osteopathic profession. Organized allopathic medicine now had a persistently difficult task in arguing the inferiority of osteopathic education. The U.S. Civil Service Commission declared in 1963 that it now recognized the DO and MD degrees as equivalent. The Department of Defense in 1966 ordered the armed forces to accept DOs into the medical corps as commissioned officers equivalent to MDs. "There was plenty of discrimination at first. I was a great guy until some of the medical officers found out I was a DO and then they would not talk to me. Some of their wives would not talk to mine. It did not matter though; I was still a captain in the United States Army Medical Corps and my performance professionally won their respect eventually."[8] The AOA was also recognized as the accreditation agency for osteopathic hospital participation in Medicare. The osteopathic profession was on the move, and the playing field was becoming more level than it had ever been in the past.

With organized osteopathic medicine enjoying its hard won achievements and no wave of mergers as was anticipated, organized allopathic medicine began to seek out other vulnerabilities of osteopathy to exploit. They had to rescind their labeling of DOs as cultists in the early 1960s for the California merger to proceed. With this label now gone, the argument could no longer be "science vs. cultism" but, instead, "better medical education vs. poorer medical education." In a series of by now bold moves, the AMA attacked osteopathic medicine's greatest vulnerability: its size. If mergers were not an option, perhaps osteopathic students, interns, and residents could be persuaded to leave for allopathic training. The AMA authorized its respective affiliated groups to allow students from osteopathic colleges to transfer into allopathic ones and to allow osteopathic graduates to enter its graduate medical education programs. It also offered national, state, and county divisional membership to DOs. Allopathic hospitals were permitted also to accept DOs for full staff privileges. Some DOs did respond, but the anticipated mass defections did not materialize. Many DOs who accepted allopathic specialty and subspeciality training returned to osteopathic hospitals and medical schools to expand the profession's residency programs and to teach.

Meanwhile, the osteopathic profession was able to use a by-product of Abraham Flexner's "reforms." A central argument of Flexner was that the health care needs of America would be better served by many fewer physicians who were better trained, more scientifically trained, in the model of Johns Hopkins. Medical schools that survived the mass closings recommended by Flexner did not increase their class sizes enough to keep pace with the growing American population. Also, allopathic medicine encouraged specialism to the point where MD general practitioners suffered in status and became outnumbered by their specialist colleagues. Specialists tend to cluster in areas of larger populations to support their practices. It became apparent by the early 1960s that America had an emerging crisis of a physician shortage and serious problems of maldistribution. Organized osteopathic medicine, with compelling data to back them up, was able to convince concerned federal and state government agencies that the profession was producing just the remedy for the problem. Osteopathic medicine had remained a generalist-oriented profession whose practitioners tended to locate proportionately into smaller communities and rural areas than did MDs.

Osteopathic medical students began to be approved on an equal basis with students of allopathic medicine and dentistry for grants and scholarships from the Health Professions Education Act (1963) and the Health Manpower Act (1968). State governments began to acknowledge the contributions of osteopathic physicians and began scholarship assistance programs to osteopathic students, as well as direct assistance to the private DO medical schools. The profession likewise continued its long tradition of self-help. Between 1961 and 1975 the Osteopathic Progress Fund provided $16 million in private donations to the schools. The colleges increased individual student tuition significantly and were finally able to provide osteopathic medical students with educational support financially equivalent with all MD medical schools. The leveling of the field economically and educationally continued to be reflected in the form of higher test scores on independent examinations. By 1972 DO scores were not statistically different than American-trained MDs on composite board examinations and remained far superior to foreign-trained physicians.[3]

Michigan Takes the Lead

Following the California merger, Michigan was thrust into the position of being the largest DO state. It now had the largest number of osteopathic physicians and the most and largest hospitals. It did not, however, have its own osteopathic medical school. The Michigan Association of Osteopathic Physicians and Surgeons (MAOPS) proposed the development of an osteopathic medical school in 1963. In a gesture very characteristic by now of self-help and self-reliance, MAOPS assessed each individual member in the state $2000 to support the effort. Political support for the DOs was very solid in Michigan because they provided generalist care that the state needed badly.

As debate raged over the possibility of state support for the school, organized osteopathic medicine saw the need for a school regardless of the legislative outcome and pressed ahead with plans to open a private medical school. The private Michigan College of Osteopathic Medicine accepted its inaugural class of 20 students in the fall of 1969. The school was established entirely from private funds. Its campus was located in Pontiac, Michigan. The push for state funding continued in the legislature, with the Michigan State Medical Society and the three MD schools in the state arguing against it at every phase. The newest of the Michigan MD programs was a 2-year school on the campus of Michigan State University that at the time was making the transition to a 4-year school. This program especially did not welcome the competition a new state-supported DO school would pose. Organized osteopathic medicine was, however, persuasive enough with the Michigan legislature to not only turn the private DO school into a public institution but to move it as well to the Michigan State University campus. Michigan State University College of Osteopathic Medicine (MSUCOM) became the first publicly funded DO medical school, as well as the first osteopathic school associated with a major university. Not withstanding the loss of its largest medical school and more than 50 years of only slow growth, the osteopathic profession rebounded in Michigan and set a major trend.[10]

Professional Expansion of Osteopathy

Shortly after the opening of MSUCOM, side-by-side with an MD school on the same campus, other large DO states used the Michigan success as their own model. In an almost identical fashion, the private Texas College of Osteopathic Medicine accepted its inaugural class in 1970. By the next year it was approved for state support, and by 1975 it came under the direction of the Board of Regents of North Texas State University. Expanding the scenario, private osteopathic medical schools in both Oklahoma and West Virginia opened in 1974 and both soon transitioned to state-supported institutions. The West Virginia school remained a free-standing medical school, but the other school became the College of Osteopathic Medicine of Oklahoma State University. Ohio and New Jersey also were to join the ranks of the state-supported osteopathic medical schools with the establishment of Ohio University College of Osteopathic Medicine and the University of Medicine and Dentistry of New Jersey School of Osteopathic Medicine, (OUCOM and UMDNJ-SOM, respectively).

The expansion continued in a number of other states with the development of both free-standing private osteopathic medical colleges and private university-based colleges of osteopathic medicine. The osteopathic profession finally received its longed-for moral and legal victory when the California Supreme Court in 1973 overturned the legislation banning DOs from being licensed in the state. This legal victory resulted in the opening of the College of Osteopathic Medicine of the Pacific in Pomona in 1978. Because osteopathic medicine provided primary-care physicians at a time when the country needed them most, the profession grew from five small private medical schools to 15 diverse colleges of osteopathic medicine in a span of 11 years. Allopathic schools expanded as well, but at a much smaller percent increase.

SUMMARY

The profession of osteopathic medicine remains a completely unique American phenomenon. It is the only one of the nineteenth century sectarian reform movements to not only survive but thrive as a parallel and distinct school of medicine. This phenomenal success has been due to a combination of factors including the expansion of the curriculum (while maintaining its central theme of the importance of the musculoskeletal system), organizational cohesiveness, political and legal savvy, and finally some extraordinary good fortune.

A part of this good fortune includes important "strategic elites," a term coined by Norman Gevitz, a sociologist. Strategic elites are those persons of stature who can speak powerfully for those not in a sufficiently powerful position to speak for themselves. Examples of this include Dr. William Smith, an academic strategic elite, the local Kirksville Presbyterian Minister, Rev. J.K. Mitchell, U.S. Senator

Foraker, local and national political strategic elites, plus many more. A sign of a profession's coming-of-age includes being noticed as a legitimate object of historical inquiry. This is where Dr. Gevitz became, perhaps unwittingly, one of the osteopathic profession's strategic elites.

In 1982 he published the book that was an outgrowth of his doctoral thesis. Gevitz's endeavor was the first dispassionate "outsider's" history of the osteopathic profession, which, even with its "warts-and-all" disclosures, nonetheless demonstrated more merit than fault. Gevitz's warning that the future of the profession is now in its own hands remains accurate and valid still. A cohort of young, bright, exquisitely well-trained osteopathic physicians are making their mark on American medicine. A large number of them have gone through their medical school experiences and graduate training isolated from the humiliating sting of prejudice common only a generation before. Prejudice still remains and the disgruntlement of those feisty former California DOs could revisit the profession with a new vigor. Issues of merger may not come from former expected quarters, but from the nonpartisan posture of the new corporate approach to health care delivery. Keeping the "reformation in progress" will mean keeping the formerly effective cohesive postures intact, but these by themselves are probably not sufficient. Osteopathic medicine will have to provide ongoing and convincing evidence that the reformation still has more to offer than its larger rival. Most DOs seem to feel that evidence is forthcoming and anticipate the playing field will continue to tilt in their direction in the foreseeable future.

Bibliography

1. Booth ER: *History of osteopathy and 20th century medical practice: osteopathic legislation,* Cincinnati, 1924, The Baxton Press.
2. Flexner A: *Medical education in the United States and Canada,* Bulletin No. 4, New York, 1910, Carnegie Foundation for the Advancement of Teaching.
3. Gevitz N: The D.O.'s: osteopathic medicine in America, Baltimore & London, 1982, The Johns Hopkins University Press.
4. Jones RM: *The Parisian education of an American surgeon: the letters of Jonathan Mason Warren,* Philadelphia, 1978, The American Philosophical Society.
5. Kaufman M: Other healers: unorthodox medicine in America. In Gevitz N (ed): *Homeopathy in America: the rise and fall and persistence of a medical heresy,* Baltimore, 1988, The Johns Hopkins University Press.
6. King LS: *The medical world of the 18th century,* Chicago, 1958, University of Chicago Press.
7. Mertiny M: *Illustrierte Geschichte der Medizin, Geschichte der Homöopathie,* Verlagsbuchhandel, Salzburg, 1986, Andreas & Andreas.
8. Osborn G: Oral history from Dr. Andrew Lovy, second osteopathic physician to receive a commission, October 1997.
9. Osborn G: Private communication: oral history from three former California D.O.'s, re: Merger, December 1997.
10. Osborn G, Mikkols, M: Oral history collected form Dr. Myron Magen, Dr. Gerald Faverman, and Mr. Thomas Angott, August 1997.
11. Osler W: *Principles & practice of medicine,* ed 8, New York, 1912, D Appleton.

12. Patent for Railroad Car switching device, Display, Still National Osteopathic Museum.
13. Professional card of A.T. Still, Archives, Still National Osteopathic Museum Kirksville, Mo.
14. Rothstein WG: *American physicians in the 19th century, from sects to science: plan of analysis,* Baltimore, 1972, The Johns Hopkins University Press.
15. Rothstein WG: Other healers. In Gevitz N: The botanical movements & orthodox medicine: eclectic medicine.
16. Starr P: *The social transformation of American medicine: The consolidation of professional authority, 1850-1930,* 1982, Basic Books.
17. Trowbridge C: *Andres Taylor Still, 1828-1917,* Kirksville, Mo, 1991, The Thomas Jefferson University Press, Northeast Missouri State University.

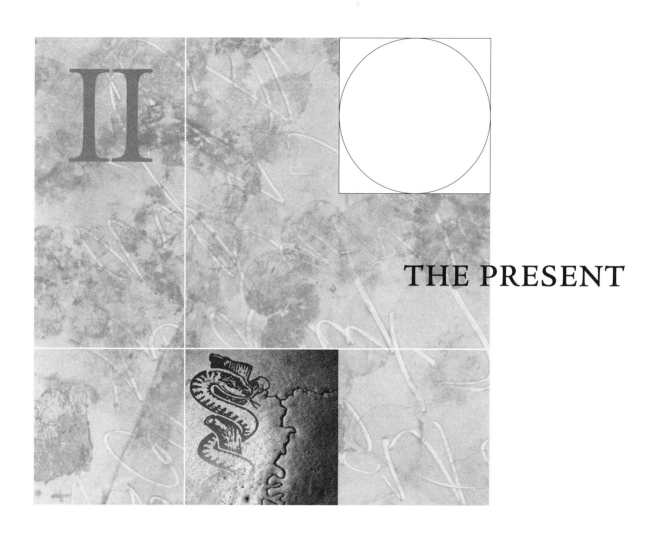

II

THE PRESENT

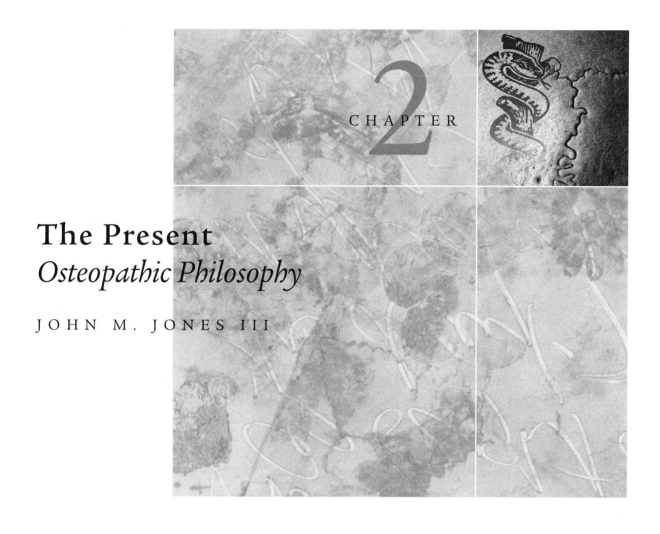

CHAPTER 2

The Present
Osteopathic Philosophy

JOHN M. JONES III

To find health should be the object of the doctor. Anyone can find disease.

ANDREW TAYLOR STILL, *Philosophy of Osteopathy*

The word *philosophy* frequently engenders an immediate visceral response in the scientific or technological mind. The scientific mind is open to processing all new ideas. The technological mind tends to reject that which has not been statistically demonstrated. Thus, the connotation of philosophy as an organization of vague or general thoughts has frequently been repugnant to the technological mind of the twentieth century. Yet some of our greatest scientists, including Einstein, spoke of the importance of thoughts that are not yet statistically evident.

In the last half of the nineteenth century, Andrew Taylor Still (Figure 2-1) developed a unified philosophy of medicine, which he called *osteopathic philosophy*. This philosophy is best described as a background reference system of ideas that

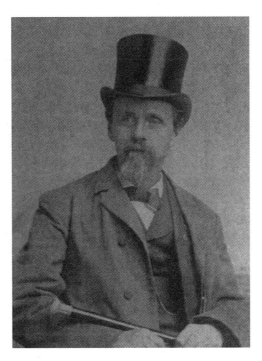

Figure 2-1 A portrait of A.T. Still, the founder of osteopathy, circa 1900. (Courtesy Kirksville College of Osteopathy, A.T. Still Memorial Library, Archives Department, Kirksville, Missouri.)

identifies the nature of the patient, establishes the physician's mission, and gives the basic premises of the logic of diagnosis and treatment. There remains in the general medical community, which has not been exposed to this organizing system, a poor understanding of exactly what is meant by osteopathic philosophy and why doctors of osteopathic medicine consider it important.

Osteopathic medical philosophy is centered around a profound respect for the inherent ability of the human being to heal itself. This philosophy has roots that go deeply through the entirety of recorded history and shares elements that were recognized by tribes of nomadic humans in prehistoric times. Over time, all new ideas evolve and are integrated with new information. Osteopathic philosophy is no exception: time has produced a distinction between classical osteopathy, which was taught by Still, and contemporary osteopathic medical philosophy, which integrates the basic elements of Still's ideas with subsequent scientific discoveries.

FOUNDING OF OSTEOPATHIC PHILOSOPHY

Andrew Taylor Still was a frontier MD whose life experience and observations led him to question the entire system of medicine that existed in nineteenth century

America. Still came to have a profound respect for the healing powers of nature. By April 1855, he stated that he began to give reasons "for my faith in the laws of life as given to men, worlds, and beings by the God of Nature. . . ."[11] He was not alone in his quest for a scientifically based philosophy of medicine. Oliver Wendell Holmes, for instance, was often quoted as saying that "if the whole *materia medica* as now used could be sunk to the bottom of the sea, it would be all the better for mankind—and all the worse for the fishes."[3,5]

The majority of medications in the nineteenth century were unresearched remedies passed on through tradition. Bleeding and leeching were major components of treatment when Still was trained. Surgery was primitive and performed without antisepsis; anesthesia was just beginning to be used. No antibiotics existed. No theory of infectious illness had been proven. There was no knowledge of the immune system. Heart disease and cancer were not understood. Physicians were, however, capable of diagnosing recognized patterns of illness and, in many cases, predicting outcomes. Medical treatment was often more dangerous than doing nothing. In fact, the famous French mathematician/philosopher Descartes, developer of the Cartesian system of thought, was reputed to have said, "Before, when I knew I was sick, I thought I might die; now that they are taking me to the chirurgeon, I know I shall."

By the time of the Civil War, a large number of American physicians were homeopathic or eclectic. In addition, many people on the frontier took care of their own medical needs. Medical education was offered in two ways. At medical school, one attended a course of 4 months of morning lectures. If one attended a second year, it was for a repeat of the same lectures. Many American physicians skipped this didactic education and apprenticed themselves to an established physician, reading medical and scientific textbooks, and accompanying the physician on his home and office visits. These two systems were later combined to give us current medical education, with 2 years of basic science and medical didactics, followed by 2 years during which students continue to read medical books and journals while shadowing and assisting physicians in hospital and ambulatory care settings.

Still had followed the standard medical practices up until the end of the Civil War in the West. In 1864, having left the Kansas Militia when the war in the west ended, he returned home. Shortly thereafter, in an epidemic of spinal meningitis, three of his children died. At this point he questioned the entirety of medical philosophy as had been taught to him. He wrote, "It was when I gazed at three members of my own family—two of my own children and one adopted child—all dead from the disease, spinal meningitis, that I propounded to myself the serious questions 'In sickness has God left man in a world of guessing? Guess what is the matter? What to give, and guess the result? And when dead, guess where he goes?'"[9]

The deaths of his children perplexed him. He also suffered a personal illness (typhoid) after this that left him with much time on his hands for thought. No doubt he recalled the time when as a teenager he had used a rope swing padded by a jacket to induce cervical traction and relieve a headache.[9] Also, his many dissections of game animals for the family food supply had shown him an incredible amount of anatomy, for which he had a deep respect. He had subsequently done much human cadaveric dissection. Included among his philosophical underpinnings were the ideas of the theory of evolution, which indicated that nature sought perfection, and the spiritual philosophy of the Methodist church, which taught that humanity should be working on attaining perfection.

His profound respect for nature led him to the conclusion that a human being was perfectly constructed. In his writings, he often refers to the God of Nature, the Great Architect, the Great Engineer, the Great Mechanic. Although he was raised with an anthropomorphic religious point of view, in his later writings he also refers to the divine source as the Unknowable. Still had a tremendous admiration for engineering and, in fact, told his students that they were to become engineers of the body. He was an inventor with a patent for a new type of churn and a stove; he had also invented a thresher.

His philosophy evolved as he continued doing dissections, treating people in as natural a way as possible, continuing to occasionally use a few of the medications common to his age. He did not know what to call what he was now doing as he developed the art of medical manipulation. For a short time he thought it had something in common with magnetic therapy, and he called himself a magnetic healer. Later his business cards indicate that he thought of himself as a lightning bonesetter. The very use of this term implies that he was aware that there were folk healers who called themselves by that name, although there is no evidence that he ever studied with anyone who had learned this art in the usual way, as it was passed from father to son.

It is questionable as to whether he had heard of the Greek physician Erisistratus, whose ideas of the profound importance of anatomy on illness had fallen to the side as Galen's elaboration of humors and disharmony in humoral balance as the etiology of disease gained precedence. However, scientists and physicians of the era were more likely to delve into Greek and Roman ideas in the 1800s than we are today, which means he may indeed have been influenced by them. He attended the Kansas City College of Medicine, but left when he felt their ideas were no better than the rest of standard contemporary medicine of the time.

It was on June 22, 1874, he says, that "I flung to the breeze the banner of Osteopathy."[9] He set up an itinerant practice of medicine in Missouri, which grew to the point where so many people came to Kirksville looking for him that he was able to settle down and stay at one office. Now some of his patients paid Still to allow them to follow him and attempt to learn this new medical art. His diagnosis was standard for the known illnesses of the time, but his conception of the etiology of illness and methods of treatment were unique. His idea was that illness had as its etiology anatomical derangement that could be detected by checking the position of the bones, primarily those of the spine, and that this affected the fluid flow in the body. Blood flow through the arteries was essential; venous and lymphatic drainage were also crucial. Axoplasmic neural flow and the flow of cerebrospinal fluid were equally important in his model of medicine.

When he founded the American School of Osteopathy in 1892 at 64 years of age, it was the first time his ideas were summarized and taught as an organized system, which he now named osteopathy. The school expanded rapidly, and it became impossible for him to personally instruct all the students in his methods. He had to depend on his initial students, who became the new professors. In order to disseminate his ideas, he wrote four books:

The Autobiography of Andrew Taylor Still (1897) describes his life and how he developed osteopathy. *The Philosophy of Osteopathy* (1899) and *The Philosophy and Mechanical Principles of Osteopathy* (copyrighted 1892 but published 1902) describe his philosophical ideas and contains a great deal of speculation about physiology, which was poorly understood at the time. But it is in *Osteopathy: Research and Practice* (1910) that he actually describes some of his treatment techniques.

These books reveal that he still, on occasion, used some medications—although extremely rarely. He was opposed to the use of opiates and alcohol, having seen much abuse (especially in Civil War victims), and specifically states that it is foolish for physicians to dissolve most medications in alcohol, as this could lead to addiction. Throughout these books he recommends the use of manipulation as an extrinsic force to relieve anatomical and therefore physiological stress on the system, returning the body to a state where it can cure itself through normal physiological processes. Still's original philosophical principles are summed up in "Our Platform," which was published in *Osteopathy: Research and Practice,* and adopted by the American School of Osteopathy as the foundation of its educational program (Box 2-1).

BOX 2-1

Our Platform

13. It should be known where osteopathy stands and what it stands for. A political party has a platform that all may know its position in regard to matters of public importance, what it stands for and what principles it advocates. The osteopath should make his position just as clear to the public. He should let the public know, in his platform, what he advocates in his campaign against disease. Our position can be tersely stated in the following planks:
14. First: We believe in sanitation and hygiene.
15. Second: We are opposed to the use of drugs as remedial agencies.
16. Third: We are opposed to vaccination.
17. Fourth: We are opposed to the use of serums in the treatment of disease. Nature furnishes its own serums if we know how to deliver them.

From Korr IM, Olgilvie CD: Health orientation in medical education, U.S. The Texas College of Osteopathic Medicine, *Prev Med* 10:710-718, 1981, Academic Press.

Continued

BOX 2-1

Our Platform—cont'd

18. Fifth: We realize that many cases require surgical treatment and therefore advocate it as a last resort. We believe many surgical operations are unnecessarily performed and that many operations can be avoided by osteopathic treatment.
19. Sixth: The osteopath does not depend on electricity, X-radiance, hydrotherapy or other adjuncts, but relies on osteopathic measures in the treatment of disease.
20. Seventh: We have a friendly feeling for other non-drug, natural methods of healing, but we do not incorporate any other methods into our system. We are all opposed to drugs; in that respect at least, all natural, unharmful methods occupy the same ground. The fundamental principles of osteopathy are different from those of any other system and the cause of disease is considered from one standpoint, viz: disease is the result of anatomical abnormalities followed by physiological discord. To cure disease the abnormal parts must be adjusted to the normal; therefore other methods that are entirely different in principle have no place in the osteopathic system.
21. Eighth: Osteopathy is an independent system and can be applied to all conditions of disease, including purely surgical cases, and in these cases surgery is but a branch of osteopathy.
22. Ninth: We believe that our therapeutic house is just large enough for osteopathy and that when other methods are brought in just that much osteopathy must move out."(6)

CLASSICAL OSTEOPATHIC PHILOSOPHY

Classical osteopathic philosophy identifies the human being as a triune being, including body, mind, and spirit. However, Still speaks very little about how to deal with the spirit or mind, leaving that up to the individual, and confines himself in general to dealing with the body of the patient. The osteopathic perspective is that the body is a marvelous machine that will function perfectly if the structure is perfect. If sick, it can be adjusted to the structural ideal to effect a return to physiological harmony. Surgery and obstetrics are included in this philosophy. Surprisingly, Still felt that the diet of his time was sufficient, and that the body (the machine) could handle any fuel as long as the machine was working right.

Still repeatedly talked about the triune nature of the human being. He frequently mentioned body, mind, and spirit. This philosophy dates back to at least the Greeks and probably the Egyptians. The body is obvious and needs no definition. The mind, however, has been described both as an epiphenomenon of the brain and its biochemistry and as something else that is more than the product of chemical interactions. Emotions are generally identified with the mind, but where the definition of the mind ends and the spirit begins is open to question. Although there are many scientists who openly question the existence of spirit, it is perhaps easiest to say that throughout history, a possible third factor of human existence has been recognized by all societies. This factor is sometimes regarded as the most potent, but the most unpredictable.

Still focused on the relationship between structure (anatomy) and function (physiology). His methods included taking a history, observation and palpation of the body, and adjustment of its constituent parts so that they were in normal positions, with normal motion, thereby promoting normal physiology. At that point, the innate self-healing powers of the body would accomplish what was necessary for healing to take place.

EVOLUTION OF THE OSTEOPATHIC PHILOSOPHY

All philosophies that survive must be capable of incorporating new information as it is discovered. Striking differences from the above original platform now exist in contemporary osteopathic medical philosophy and practice.

Still died in 1917. By 1911 the American School of Osteopathy (ASO) had incorporated the teaching of vaccines, serum therapy, and antitoxins in the bacteriology course.[12] Also by 1911 the first modern antibiotic, the arsenical compound Salvarsan, which had been developed by Paul Erlich, had been successfully used against syphilis *(Treponema pallidum)*.[8] The development of antibiotics derived from the study of tissue by pathologists, who first noted that tissue could be stained by certain chemicals that affected only particular cells. This generated the idea that it would be possible to develop a chemical that was toxic to infectious microbes but would spare the body's cells. After Salvarsan, the sulfa drugs were developed by the 1930s. As new medicines were developed and researched, the faculty and students at the ASO adopted the teaching of *materia medica* (that aspect of medical science concerned with the origin and preparation of drugs, their doses, and their mode of administration) in 1928. Prior to this, many students had studied pharmacology informally with some of the professors who were MDs.

By the 1930s, the osteopathic philosophy had been expanded to include medicines that had proven their value through research, as illustrated in this introductory quote from the 1935 edition of the *Sage Sayings of Still:*

> Osteopathy is not a drugless therapy in the strict sense of the word. It uses drugs which have specific scientific value, such as antiseptics, parasiticides, antidotes, anesthetics or narcotics for the temporary relief of suffering. It is the empirical internal administration of drugs for therapeutic purposes that osteopathy opposes, substituting instead manipulation, mechanical measures and the balancing of the life essentials as more rational and more in keeping with the physiological functions of the body. The osteopathic physician is the skilled engineer of the vital human mechanism, influencing by manipulation and other osteopathic measures the activities of the nerves, cells, glands and organs, the distribution of fluids and the discharge of nerve impulses, thus normalizing tissue, fluid and function.[13]

Antiseptic surgical technique was developed at about the same time as the development of osteopathy, and this was included in surgical procedures practiced by the new profession. One difference between the allopathic and osteopathic approaches was that patients received osteopathic manipulative treatment before and after surgery. Postsurgical treatment focused on soft tissue and rib raising, an articulatory treatment designed to increase the efficiency of breathing while calming down the sympathetic nervous system.

The development of the sulfa antibiotics, along with their more common usage in hospital cases in the 1930s, and the advent of penicillin (developed in 1927 but not commercially available until after World War II in 1945) significantly changed the practice of all medicine. Except for a very few older physicians who felt manipulation was the only answer, osteopathic physicians adopted these miracle medicines immediately. It was with the integration of medicines that were researched and effective that classic osteopathic philosophy expanded to a more comprehensive contemporary osteopathic medical philosophy.

Following the evolution of osteopathic thought, George W. Northup, DO, was quoted as saying:

> It is now better understood that a given 'disease' is not so easily defined as was once believed. The search for a single cause for a single disease has produced disillusionment. Even the 'germ theory' is not sufficient to provide a 'simple' explanation for infectious diseases. All of us live in a world of potential bacterial invasion, but relatively few become infected. There are multiple causes, even in bacterially induced diseases. Disease is a total body response. It is not merely a stomach ulcer, a broken bone, or a troublesome mother-in-law. It is a disturbance of the structure-function of the body and not an isolated or local insult. Equally important is the recognition that disease is multicausal. The understanding that multiple causes of disease can arise from remote but interconnected parts of the body will ultimately emerge into a unifying philosophy for all of medicine. When this occurs, it will embrace many of the basic principles of osteopathic medicine."[7]

The shift in osteopathic thought embraced the progress of the scientific development of medicine in the twentieth century, but maintained the belief that it is not the physician who heals, but the body itself, which heals through its homeostatic mechanisms. Contemporary osteopathic medical philosophy also maintains a belief in the efficacy of manipulation to decrease physiological and sometimes psychological stress, therefore assisting the body to regain optimal homeostatic levels.

Still's original opposition to the medicine of his time is seen as the product of the lack of research on the medicines that were used. One of his better known quotes is that "Man should study and use the drugs compounded in his own body."[9] This is increasingly the method of study today: finding out how the body works and then using medicines that interact with the body's cellular receptors and that mimic the compounds found in the body or, in some cases, that are identical to compounds found in the body.

CONTEMPORARY DIFFERENCES WITH "OUR PLATFORM"

Addressing each of the planks of the platform, today's osteopathic physicians would have the following comments.

- Hygienic and sanitary measures have, in fact, decreased mortality and morbidity in modern society far more than other medical measures.

- Much of Still's criticism of the medicine of his day was provoked precisely because it was not researched and therefore, to him, without logic and not scientifically valid. However, there have been only a very few osteopathic physicians, most of them at the end of the nineteenth or beginning of the twentieth century, who were completely opposed to all medicines. Contemporary medications are often overused, resulting in a higher annual number of deaths due to medication side effects than from highway accidents.

- Immunization is now achieved with standard purified doses and is much better understood. Statistics have demonstrated that the morbidity and mortality rates associated with not using immunizations are considerably worse than those found when immunizations are used. Although it is impossible to predict the outcome of immunization in an individual case, (and some react to the medium), the patient who succumbs to an idiosyncratic reaction to a vaccine may be the one who would have had a similar reaction to the disease in an epidemic if the population were not immunized.

- Serums or other blood parts in Still's day were much more dangerous than those found today. However, AIDS and other blood-borne diseases have demonstrated that body fluids, cell and cell parts must be used with appropriate caution.

- Surgery is overused in the United States, but the medical community is working on the development of more conservative approaches, and the use of aseptic technique, improved anesthesia, microscopic and endoscopic surgery has diminished many negative consequences.

- All therapies that are statistically demonstrated to aid patients are completely acceptable. Still was apparently never opposed to the use of x-rays for diagnostic purposes, since the ASO had the second diagnostic x-ray machine west of the Mississippi River. The use of radiation therapy as we know it was unknown in his time, as was the use of lasers for therapeutic purposes.

- We recognize that disease has multiple etiologies that were unknown in Still's day (e.g., genetic abnormality, nutritional deficiencies, psychosomatic effects) and that his unifactorial description of the etiology of illness is no longer tenable. The therapeutic house of the osteopathic profession, except for a few of its founding members, has always included the latest of research on medications and the expansion in medical knowledge through this past century. However, the incorporation of this expanded knowledge into medical school curricula has resulted in less available instructional time for osteopathic manipulation, leaving some physicians less skilled and neglecting its use in appropriate cases.

Contemporary Osteopathic Medical Philosophy

As we enter the twenty-first century, we find the following official definition of the term *osteopathic philosophy* in the "Glossary of Osteopathic Terminology" section of the AOA Yearbook, 2000[1]:

> Osteopathic philosophy: Osteopathic medicine is a philosophy of health care and a distinctive art, supported by expanding scientific knowledge; its philosophy embraces the concept of the unity of the living organism's structure (anatomy) and function (physiology). Its art is the application of the philosophy in the practice of medicine and surgery in all its branches and specialties. Its science includes the behavioral, chemical, physical, spiritual and biological knowledge related to the establishment and maintenance of health as well as the prevention and alleviation of disease.

Osteopathic concepts emphasize the following principles[1]:
1. The human being is a dynamic unit of function.
2. The body possesses self-regulatory mechanisms which are self-healing in nature.
3. Structure and function are interrelated at all levels.
4. Rational treatment is based on these principles.

Contemporary osteopathic medical philosophy begins with classical osteopathy and integrates additional knowledge. Rather than applying the choice either/or to manipulation or medicine, both/and is frequently appropriate. Other evolved changes include recently developed knowledge of nutrition, exercise, environmental factors, genetics, and psychology.

For instance, nutrition is considered important. Still had not considered it important, and often recommended that the patients just "eat what they want of good plain nutritious food."[9] The reason nutritional importance was added into the philosophy was that in the time of Still, all crops were grown organically, and most of the population of the United States was in a rural environment. Although he mentions good food several times, he assumed that the average diet in those times was sufficient for nourishment, as opposed, for instance, to Graham, who invented what he thought was the ideal food, the Graham cracker. In Still's time, the importance of vitamins and trace minerals, as well as the importance of macronutrient balance (protein, carbohydrates, fats) had not been elaborated.

For exercise, Still occasionally mentioned walking or horseback riding. In the preautomotive society, there was little need to recommend these: everyone in America walked or rode horseback to get where they were going. A great many laborsaving devices had not been invented, so normal daily living took care of most of the exercise needs of the population.

Likewise, the dangers of excessive solar radiation to health had not yet become apparent in a society in which tanning was not considered attractive. Farmers often wore long-sleeve shirts and hats, and even swimsuits provided practically full clothing of the body and often were paired with a parasol for protection from the sun. Air pollution, water pollution, and noise pollution were not considered as causes of illness, nor were workplace toxins. Radiation damage was unheard of, and the immune system undiscovered, although Still's works are replete with references to the body's capacity to maintain health, particularly with an open arterial conduit providing a good blood supply to the tissues.

Genetic mutations/deficiencies also were unknown. Physicians were virtually ignorant of the science of genetics at the end of the nineteenth century. Current research promises multiple benefits from our expanding knowledge of molecular biology. This knowledge has great potential for both good and harm. Its application will also fit in well with osteopathic philosophy.

Mind/body approaches have shown considerable development for patient applications. Biofeedback and the *relaxation response* have been validated by research as ways of manipulating homeostatic values to improve immune system parameters. Psychological counseling techniques have advanced the possibilities for patients to address the stresses in their psychosocial milieu.

All of these etiological factors of illness have therefore been integrated into an expanded contemporary osteopathic philosophy while retaining the profound respect for the ability of the body to function in the face of many challenges and its inherent capacity for self-healing when injury or illness is present.

Whereas Still thought the body was basically perfect as it was and could process environmental and nutritional input without damage unless there was an injury that gave structural damage. We now know that the human being is continuous with the environment, and on more than one level (body: physical, mind: thought/emotion, spirit: emotion/beliefs/other subtle factors). Illness is seen by the twenty-first century osteopathic physician as having multiple etiologies, any one of which can be the initiator or promoter. Nonetheless, all of these factors potentially affect the structure of the body, whether at a gross (neuromusculoskeletal) level or at a microscopic (stereochemical/bioelectrochemical) level.

Wellness therefore lies along a continuum with illness, across the timeframe between the points of conception and death. Illness begins as wellness decreases. Wellness indicates that the individual is capable of accepting multiple challenges without homeostasis declining to the point of interference with normal activities. As the system loses optimal homeostatic balance, less of an environmental/mental insult is needed to precipitate a state of illness.

Early in the continuum lie such problems as nutritional deficiency, insufficient exercise or rest, and inappropriate levels of stress. If these problems are addressed while they are simple, the organism recovers and retains adaptability. On an overlapping/interactive continuum lies the problem of gross structural integrity, involving bilateral muscle tone balance, and neural activity levels, especially in the autonomic nervous system, and particularly as these factors affect the respiratory, circulatory, lymphatic, endocrine, and immune systems.

Simple problems can sometimes be solved by the use of manipulation, lifestyle changes (e.g., exercises) or nutrition in order to reestablish optimal homeostatic set points. When nothing is done, our homeostatic mechanisms may effect a recovery without aid. Sometimes the body does not have the ability to recover on its own. In such a case, either gross or microscopic level structural dysfunction can be compounded by the sequelae of inflammation, pain, and tissue congestion. These negative changes in the biochemical environment of the body can cause many variables in the endocrine and immune systems to swing to wider extremes and destabilize one or more of the body's systems, leading to illness.

Ideas such as these are not easily understood by a reductionistic approach to the body, in which each variable is analyzed by itself or perhaps in conjunction with one or two other variables (e.g., insulin and glucagon). Current understanding recognizes much more complexity in interaction between many more subtle variables, such as eicosanoids, the biochemicals that control many body functions and that evolved before bipolar hormonal control systems.

Chaos mathematical analysis and fractal analysis have enabled greater understanding of the complexity of dynamical medical systems. Chaos mathematics allows us to understand how affecting a single, or even a few variables in one system (e.g., cardiovascular) can affect the function of other systems, and thereby the entire human being. One factor that has been noted is the phenomenon known as "sensitive dependence on initial conditions," or the butterfly effect, which indicates that a simple motion such as that of a butterfly's wings in New York may affect the weather patterns in Moscow 3 months later.[4] Although this is an example that makes us chuckle, the mathematical models following chaos principles appear to be closer to what happens in the natural world than any previous analysis. Mathematicians are working on models of such things as the decompensating cycle of cardiac arrhythmia to fatal fibrillation.[4] Understanding such new concepts as point attractors, strange attractors, triviality, nontriviality, and degeneracy leads to a better understanding of the processes of homeostasis and how manipulation of anatomical parameters and tissue tensions can promote physiological adaptability.

Each system is understood to be an avenue of access to the entire body, to the person. The neuromusculoskeletal system can be considered the largest single system in the body, one that reflects the state of health of the other systems, thereby yielding diagnostic clues for systemic or organic function/dysfunction. It can also be used as an access for treatment, through the use of manipulation to change the set points of muscle tone, thereby affecting vascular and lymphatic flow as well as neural (particularly autonomic) tone.

THE SECOND GREAT OSTEOPATHIC PHILOSOPHER: IRVIN KORR, PHD

Irvin Korr, PhD, is perhaps the second best known osteopathic philosopher in the past hundred years. Andrew Taylor Still spoke often of the importance of structure (anatomy) and function (physiology), but largely confined his studies to anatomy, medical diagnosis, and osteopathic treatment. Physiology in the late 1800s and the beginning of the twentieth century was largely speculative. By the 1940s, Sted Denslow, DO, was heading a research program at Kirksville to investigate the physiology of the osteopathic lesion (somatic dysfunction). He recruited Irvin Korr, whose degree in physiology was to prove crucial to this work. Korr spent 30 years doing physiological research at Kirksville, working with Denslow and other osteopathic physicians who diagnosed and treated the research subjects.

Korr and Denslow demonstrated changes in the sympathetic nervous system at levels of somatic dysfunction related to spinal segments, diagnosed by palpation. Korr sought to explain the initiation and maintenance of somatic dysfunction through studies of mechanoreceptors and proprioceptors, including the muscle spindles. He and Denslow theorized that a segment of the spinal cord could become facilitated, causing an increased response by muscles, nerves, blood vessels, and other anatomical structures at a decreased threshold level. This produced a model that described the tissue texture abnormalities, static asymmetries, restriction of motion, and tenderness that osteopathic physicians were able to palpate when diagnosing the patient. Korr was also nominated for the Nobel Prize for being the first to demonstrate axonal transport of proteins from the central nervous system to the muscles helping to explain why muscle atrophy occurs when nerves are cut or damaged.

Korr received his PhD from Princeton, where he also did postgraduate work before joining the faculty of the New York University School of Medicine in physiology. During World War II, he participated in war research for the Department of Defense at several locations before going to Kirksville in late 1945 after the war was over. He was to remain in Kirksville for 30 years.

In 1975 he went to Michigan State University, College of Osteopathic Medicine for 3 years, leaving in 1978 to work at Texas College of Osteopathic Medicine (University of North Texas Health Science Center in Fort Worth). In this last position, from which he retired at 80 (as the oldest state employee) in 1989, he published significant articles on osteopathic medical philosophy and its potential for application in contemporary medicine.

Korr continually stressed Still's philosophy that health comes from within the person, meaning that our efforts as physicians should focus on prevention.[6] He spoke of homeostatic mechanisms as the body's own health maintenance organization (HMO). Reminding us that we cannot implement our thoughts without using the neuromusculoskeletal system, he referred to it as our primary system.

The internal organs are often thought of as primary to life (particularly the heart and brain), but in truth, neither this argument nor any other action can occur without using the musculoskeletal system. Our other organ systems serve to support our musculoskeletal activities, through which we turn our thoughts into action. This is another way of stating what Still referred to as the law of mind, matter, and motion.

Korr showed that the osteopathic lesion, now renamed somatic dysfunction, served as a neurological lens for the body. His experiments demonstrated that a stimulus at a particular spinal cord level would actually give a more pronounced response at the level of dysfunction than at the level of the stimulus. Other musculoskeletal stimuli, as well as psychological stimuli (demonstrated in medical students), also focus a higher level response at the facilitated segment, therefore causing the dysfunctional segment to act as a lens. This lens can focus additional negative effects on neurologically related structures.

Holistic Models of Human Physiological Function and Dysfunction

In 1987, the Educational Council on Osteopathic Principles (composed of OMM departmental chairs from the [then] 15 osteopathic medical colleges) produced a document called the *Core Curriculum for Osteopathic Education* for the American Association of Colleges of Osteopathic Medicine (AACOM) Council of Deans. Six models of systemic function and dysfunction were included in this outline, all of which are recognized as playing a role in health.

- The *biomechanical-neuromusculoskeletal model* focuses on stress-related neuromuscular patterns that are apparent as altered posture, motion, and gait; states that biomechanical compensatory mechanisms induce segmental facilitation; and notes that associated ligamentous weakening and connective tissue disturbances often lead to irreversible joint and postural changes.
- The *neurological model* emphasizes facilitated states in the spinal cord, sympathicotonia, reflex mechanisms, trophic function of nerves, the effects and importance of pain, and behavioral response to stressors as a suprasegmental factor (influence of the brain on spinal cord-neuromusculoskeletal functions).
- The *behavioral model* emphasizes that illness is the behavioral aspect of a disease process, and that there is an interactive relationship between illness, behavior, and disease processes (the biopsychosocial spectrum of the behavioral model). Disease can be initiated by behavior (e.g., smoking) as well as causing secondary effects on the person (e.g., depression).
- The *energy expenditure and exchange model* states that the more efficient the body is, the less energy it wastes, and that this is important because energy conservation improves adaptability to stressors (through increased homeo-

static adaptive reserve). Optimal energy exchange is therefore a basic thermodynamic principle behind maintaining maximal homeostatic adaptive responses.

- The *nutritional model* reminds us that deficiencies and excesses of macronutrients (carbohydrates, proteins, and fats; fiber and water) and micronutrients (vitamins, minerals) have effects on biochemical processes and can disrupt cellular functions. Reciprocal relationships exist between nutritional requirements, cellular and systemic functions, infectious processes, drug interactions, and lifestyle stressors. Nutrition has a direct and an indirect influence on the neuromusculoskeletal system. Nutritional factors therefore act as stressors and potentiators of adaptive responses. With the change of the average American diet over the past 100 years, this has attained increased significance.

- With the *respiratory-circulatory model,* we note that altered respiratory mechanisms often predispose parts of the body to congestive changes, decreased lymphatic flow, and venous return with consequent edema formation. Vascular compromise is seen as a significant pathological factor in the disease process, and the microscopic effects of somatic dysfunction (edema and inflammation) predispose the body to altered physiological and systemic dysfunction.

In summary, each of these models is founded on the assumption that reduction and breakdown of adaptive capabilities creates pathophysiological processes, with disease being viewed as a dysfunction in the body's capacity to respond effectively to stressors.[3] Osteopathic diagnosis and treatment attempts to assess and influence the adaptive resources available to an individual at any particular moment. The physician should bear in mind all of these models, each of which focuses on an aspect of the human being's interactive functional processes.

GENERAL OSTEOPATHIC PRINCIPLES

Osteopathic principles are commonsense ideas to an osteopathic physician, which serve as a milieu in which to diagnose and treat a patient. Here we will consider a series of ideas on how to approach a patient and a list of osteopathic aphorisms. At some level, always be aware of the following:

Who is the patient? The patient is a human being like ourselves, a functional unity of body (a genetically constructed grouping of cells and systems), mind (thoughts/emotions), and a third factor (identified by some as spirit), which is interactive with the environment at physical, psychosocial, and energetic levels. The human being functions by transforming thought into action through the musculoskeletal system.

Where does health arise? Health comes from within.

What is the goal of the osteopathic physician? Seek health in the patient. Wellness and illness exist on a continuum, or on an interactive multidimensional group of continuua. Seek the highest possible level of homeostatic balance and performance within the limitations of the individual patient and the current circumstances.

How do we seek health in the patient? Prevention is the best medicine; we encourage and teach the patients to follow healthful practices (appropriate rest, nutrition, exercise, breathing, thoughts/emotions, relaxation, social interaction), and avoid that which is self-destructive (tobacco, radiation, toxins, excessive alcohol, drugs).

If the patient has entered the illness end of the continuum, we must take a careful history, perform a physical examination, and formulate a differential diagnosis, including all standard diagnostic medical practices. As we do so, we use the musculoskeletal system as an access point for diagnostic indicators (and later, for imparting information to the other systems). Tests may be needed. After arriving at a diagnosis, we decide on necessary treatment, bearing in mind all factors that affect the physiology/performance of the patient.

What factors affect the physiology of the patient? Physiology can be affected by air, water, and food; nutritional supplements; prescription or over-the-counter medications; physical forces and impacts on the system (from the effects of any movement, including exercise, to trauma); thoughts, emotions, stress, or relaxation; and energy (from gravity to sunlight to magnetic field to energies of which we may not yet be aware). All of the body's systems are integrative, but five are more easily seen as unifying systems of global communication (cardiovascular/lymphatic, respiratory, neurological, endocrine, immune systems).

The host has control of vulnerability to illness through the immune system and homeostatic mechanisms *(vis medicatrix naturae)*. When host control decreases and the system downgrades into illness, intervention is necessary. Our intervention is designed to support a system that is no longer functioning at an appropriately high level of homeostasis.

How do we intervene? Wellness, injury, and illness exist along a continuum; so do treatment approaches. Where physical or emotional force has deranged anatomical/physiological performance, we address the problems with physical approaches, ranging from manipulation to surgery. Where genetic limitations or illness make it impossible for the body to perform appropriate functions on its own, or with the speed required, we use exogenous substances such as nutritional supplementation, medication, or appropriate genetic therapy. (From the point of view of chaos mathematics and dynamical systems, we seek to reverse abnormal trivial point attractors to strange attractor status.) We do this in a conservative manner, bearing in mind the body's innate intelligence and the wisdom of making the least possible intervention (least invasive) for the greatest possible results.

BOX 2-2

Osteopathic Aphorisms

Every osteopathic physician recalls the arduous and challenging road through medical school and postgraduate training. It seemed at times to be a never-ending, rocky climb, punctuated by the ringing in our ears of our instructors' sage words. Most of the following statements are unique to the osteopathic branch of medical training.
  Seek health in your patient. (Still)
  First, do no harm. (Hippocrates)
  You will cure nothing; *the patient* will cure himself. You will attempt to assist this process.
  The artery rules supreme. (Still)
  The CSF is in command. (Still)
  Lymph is life.
  We strike at life and death when we hunt in the fascia. (Still)
  The law of mind, matter and motion. (Still)
  Address the autonomics.
  Diaphragms act as horizontal baffles in an otherwise longitudinal fluid system.
  Whenever you do osteopathic manipulative treatment (OMT), have these priorities:
    Safety of the patient
    Safety of the physician
    Efficacy of the treatment
    Ergonomics (energy efficiency for the physician giving the treatment)
  Local manipulation can have global effects.
  Global manipulation can have local effects.
  Choose endogenous solutions over exogenous solutions whenever possible.

OSTEOPATHIC TECHNIQUES

Osteopathy is not a system of techniques, but a philosophy that is often applied through techniques of osteopathic manipulative medicine, most of which were developed by osteopathic physicians. Because of interest in what these techniques may be, several of the more commonly recognized osteopathic diagnosis and treatment systems are described here. There are, of course, many others. These techniques exist along a continuum of effect, one logically leading to another, depending on the problem of the patient and the perception and skill of the osteopathic physician.

It has been said that there are only two types of techniques, direct and indirect. Direct treatment is treatment that confronts restriction of motion, in which the body part is taken in the direction of restriction. Indirect treatment is treatment in which the body part is taken in the direction of ease of motion. Once the body part is appropriately positioned, activating forces are applied to induce changes in muscle tone; central, peripheral or autonomic nervous system tone; (level of activation); and vascular/lymphatic response. The goals of treatment include tissue relaxation, increased physiological motion, decrease in pain, and optimization of homeostasis. The following are some of the more common systems of osteopathic manipulative treatment (OMT). It should be stated that manipulation of any form has both indications and contraindications; these are not discussed here, as they are well outlined in other texts.

Soft Tissue and Lymphatic Treatments

Soft tissue treatment, generally a direct treatment, was developed by Still and his early students and is sometimes confused with massage. The techniques focus on altering the tone of muscle and connective tissue. Soft tissue treatment increases arterial delivery, relaxes muscles and connective tissue, and alters the tone of the autonomic nervous system, whereas lymphatic techniques focus on increasing lymphatic and venous drainage.

High Velocity, Low Amplitude Thrust

In the direct method of treatment referred to as high velocity, low amplitude (HVLA) thrust, the restrictive barrier is engaged by precise positioning of the body. The thrust when the body part is at the restrictive barrier is very rapid (high velocity) but operates over a very short distance (low amplitude), gapping the articulation by perhaps ⅛ inch. This allows a reset of both joint position and muscle tension levels, which will cause related neural and vascular readjustment.

Articulatory Technique

The original general articulatory technique, developed by Still and his students, takes the body part being treated through the end portion of its restricted range of motion in a gentle, repetitive fashion. The repeated articulation directly diminishes the restrictive barrier. One or more planes or motion are treated at a time. This treatment can be used to treat either individual joints or regions (e.g., cervical spine, shoulder).

Still also used specific articulation techniques which began with diagnosis, placing the body parts in the direction of ease of motion, and rotating them into the direction of restriction. It is these specific articulation techniques which have been called *Still Technique* (van Buskirk). *Facilitated Positional Release* (Schiowitz) is a variation of these specific articulation techniques that Still developed.

Muscle Energy

Muscle energy was developed by Fred Mitchell, Sr., DO. It is most commonly used as a direct treatment, and the term *muscle energy* means that the patient will use his or her own energy through directed muscular cooperation with the physician. Voluntary isometric contraction of a patient's muscle(s) is followed by a gentle stretch of the dysfunctional, contracted muscle(s), decreasing abnormal restriction of motion. Other muscle energy techniques employ traction on the muscle to pull an articulation back into appropriate position.

Counterstrain Technique

Counterstrain is a passive positional technique that places the patient's dysfunctional joint (spinal or other) or tissue in a position of ease. This position arrests the inappropriate proprioceptive activity that maintains the somatic dysfunction. Marked shortening of the involved muscle or connective tissue is maintained for 90 seconds. An inappropriate strain reflex (a result of injury) is therefore inhibited by application of a counterstrain. Diagnosis is primarily by palpation of areas of tenderness mapped by the originator of this system, Lawrence Jones, DO. This form of diagnosis can also be integrated with positional or movement changes. The tender point is indicative of inappropriate neurological balance. This system is ideal for the patient who does not respond well to articulatory techniques, such as the postsurgical patient.

Myofascial Release

Myofascial release is actually a renaming of original osteopathic techniques developed by Still, which were called fascial techniques by the early osteopathic physicians. Anthony Chila, Robert Ward, and John Peckham developed a course in these techniques at Michigan State University, in which they also acknowledged the importance of the muscle tissue to the treatment. This technique may be performed in a direct or indirect manner and involves either shortening the contracted tissue (indirect) or lengthening it (direct) and allowing the nervous and respiratory systems to direct changes. Two physiological biomechanical tissues processes, creep and hysteresis, also play a role. Compression, traction, and/or respiratory cooperation can be included to facilitate the treatment.

Osteopathy in the Cranial Field (OCF, Cranial, Craniosacral)

This technique has been known by all of the above names, and was developed by William G. Sutherland, DO. It is usually done as a mixture of indirect and direct procedures, which work with the body's inherent rhythmic motions. It is commonly used in adults as a treatment for headaches or temporomandibular joint (TMJ) dysfunction syndrome and in infants (where the skull is more flexible) for treatment of symptoms related to cranial nerve compression (vomiting, poor sleep, poor feeding). Although cranial techniques focus on the skull and the sacrum, where the dura mater also attaches, they can be used throughout the body.

Visceral Techniques

A variety of techniques have been developed from the beginning of the profession to address imbalance in the viscera. These include stretching and balancing techniques related to ligamentous attachments (Still) and may involve use of inherent visceral motion.

EXAMPLES OF DIAGNOSIS AND TREATMENT IN OSTEOPATHY

Osteopathic diagnosis and treatment are determined by the osteopathic philosophy, making the practice of osteopathic medicine distinctive and different. This philosophy, and osteopathic manipulative treatment, are not merely the addition of something extra to the contemporary Western medical approach (the cherry on top of the ice cream sundae). The philosophy serves as an organizer of thought that helps the physician understand what is going on in the entire organism, allows concurrent reductionistic analysis, and then reassembles the parts into the totality of the human being (who is more than the sum of the parts).

The diagnosis differs in that the osteopathic physician does a standard physical examination, but also includes palpation and motion testing in the musculoskeletal system that is different from the standard orthopedic examination. The musculoskeletal system serves as an access point for additional diagnostic information, not only on muscle tension, but on fluid distribution and autonomic levels of activity. Well-known neurological interactions permit a physician to conclude from musculoskeletal evidence that an underlying visceral problem may exist and should be investigated.

Four criteria are used to diagnose somatic dysfunction: tissue texture abnormalities, static or positional asymmetry, restriction of motion, and tenderness. These have been referred to by the diagnostic mnemonic TART or sometimes STAR (with "sensitivity" replacing "tenderness.") At spinal segment levels where these are noted, the knowledge of reflex relationships guides the osteopathic physician to pay more attention to both the history and physical examination of the internal organs related to that spinal cord segmental level. The examination therefore includes the concept of viscerosomatic, somatovisceral, viscerovisceral and somatosomatic reflexes. These are related to accompanying autonomic nervous system influence at that level is also involved in the tissue texture changes and affects muscle tone.

Treatment is also affected by this philosophy. If the nervous system and musculoskeletal system can be used for diagnosis, it is also true that an attempt may be made to reverse pathophysiology by treating the affected anatomical structures to change their physiological performance (decreasing, for instance, inappropriate sympathetic nervous system tone and thereby enhancing homeostatic balance and adaptability). Medication or surgery may be unnecessary, depending on the severity of the problem. Osteopathic manipulative treatment (OMT) may be used as a primary means of treatment for a problem that appears to be of a nonsevere, musculoskeletal origin, or as adjunctive therapy along with medication or surgery—again, to enhance homeostatic recovery and adaptability.

Two simple examples of cases are given below. These are not complete cases, but are designed to illustrate some of the osteopathic differences in approach to diagnosis and treatment.

Case Example 1

A 67-year-old black female with a 30 pack/year history of smoking presents at the office with a productive cough that she has had for 2 weeks. She now has a fever, and the sputum is greenish in color. She has pain in the ribs on the left side of the thorax, and audible rhonchi when examined with the stethoscope. After a careful history and physical examination, the physician concludes that although the differential diagnosis includes a possible tumor, this is less likely than a community-acquired pneumonia. Radiographic studies indicate a left lingular pneumonitis, and there is an increased WBC count with a left shift. The physician has noted on examination that pulmonary viscerosomatic reflexes are activated in the corresponding thoracic spinal region, causing limitation in range of motion and tenderness, along with tissue texture changes, at several thoracic vertebral segments. Several ribs on the left have diminished mobility, and the diaphragm has decreased excursion on the left.

The physician decides to start antibiotics immediately, and treats the thoracic segments and ribs with OMT, in this case choosing counterstrain because no muscular effort is required of the patient, and there is minimal risk of injury to bones that may be osteoporotic. In patients who are coughing frequently, breathing mechanics are often disturbed. Treating the thoracic segments and ribs helps normalize the sympathetic nervous system activity and increase the efficiency and ease of breathing. The thoracic outlet, where the thoracic lymphatic duct has passage, is treated, allowing for less tissue compression to impede flow of lymphatic fluid. The diaphragm (often having impaired motion from the spasmodic motion of coughing) is treated with myofascial release, and the cervical region is treated with counterstrain to decrease any problems with the phrenic nerve (which innervates the diaphragm for respiration), and a lymphatic pump concludes the treatment. Antitussives are prescribed along with the antibiotics and an expectorant. Acetaminophen may be used for fever and pain. The patient is seen again in 3 days, at which time she is greatly improved.

The rationale behind the medical treatment is obvious: kill the bacteria, decrease the viscosity of the mucus that holds them so they can be coughed out, and give the patient a painkiller to decrease pain. This type of treatment relies on the body to recover its optimal performance once certain negatives are cancelled out. The osteopathic treatment is designed to aid normal physiological processes that augment the body's natural systems in killing the bacteria and reducing pain. The effect is to enhance the positives, not just cancel the negative effects on physiology. Even if no medicine were available, this might be enough to enable a faster recovery for the patient—or allow survival. Clearly, however, the osteopathic physician takes advantage of both possibilities, aiding the host's natural defenses while at the same time fighting the bacteria directly. The patient's comfort level is also increased by the use of the osteopathic manipulation. ∾

Case Example 2

A 19-year-old white male college student presents with an apparent sprained ankle. The injury occurred during a soccer game when he reached for the ground with his foot and made a sudden turn. There is no other relevant history. The ankle is swollen, and the patient applied ice immediately after the injury. He can walk, but keeps most of his weight off the ankle. There is pinpoint tenderness at the posteroinferior right lateral malleolus.

The physician chooses to treat with superficial indirect myofascial release and afterward, lymphatic techniques to decrease the edema. Treatment is specifically limited to a minimal approach, which causes the patient no pain. The patient is given a set of crutches to use for a couple of days and goes to the hospital to get an x-ray study, which is negative. He is to use ice at least 3 times a day and to keep his weight off the ankle, which is wrapped after the treatment with an elastic bandage. He is to keep the ankle elevated when possible, and to use acetaminophen for pain if needed. When the study shows no fracture, the physician continues the treatment 2 days later with counterstrain and lymphatic treatment, and the patient is allowed to discontinue the crutches.

Acetaminophen does not help the healing process directly. However, draining excess fluid and decreasing the overabundance of proinflammatory neuropeptides and other biochemicals through the use of OMT allows the hypertonic and injured tissues to return to normal more quickly. The decrease or elimination of muscle spasm allows the ankle and foot to have more normal mechanics, therefore promoting more normal lymphatic and venous drainage. Again, the osteopathic treatment is designed to enhance the body's own methods of healing, promoting a rapid return to more normal homeostatic balance by removing dysfunction. ∾

In both of these examples, the techniques chosen did not challenge the patients with muscular effort and were selected with homeostatic effects in mind (decrease of edema, mobilization of fluids, enhancement of respiration). In many other ambulatory cases, any of the listed treatments could be selected (such as HVLA thrust), based on four factors: the condition of the patient, the nature of the complaint, the goals of treatment, and the skills of the physician.

WHY IS MANIPULATION A CRITICAL ASPECT OF OSTEOPATHIC PHILOSOPHY?

If osteopathy is a philosophy, then why is the use of manipulation in the practice of medicine considered its hallmark and a necessary, integral part of osteopathic medicine? The answer lies in the original osteopathic philosophy, which relates to the interaction between structure (anatomy) and function (physiology) in the human species, and how we can effect changes in the human body. It can be found at two levels, the macroscopic and the microscopic.

At the macroscopic level, it is easy to see that if we have abnormal pressure on a joint, nerve, or blood vessel, there may be changes in tissue as a result over a period of time. For instance, if there is more pressure on the medial aspect of the right knee, over a period of time there will be changes in the cartilage and bone to compensate. There will also be changes in the gait as the body attempts to balance itself in the best equilibrium possible to use the least amount of energy for posture and gait. Thus, local dysfunction can induce global dysfunction. Manipulation, which has local effects of adjusting the balance in the musculoskeletal system, therefore also has global effects at a gross level.

At a microscopic level, we must analyze cellular physiology. The original one-celled organisms were bathed in a solution of seawater, which contained needed oxygen and nutrients, and which also took away toxic waste products and carbon dioxide as they were produced and ejected from the cell. Multicellular organisms such as the human being contain an internal ocean with the same functions. This internal fluid system is the cardiovascular system, delivering oxygen and nutrients to each individual cell, clearing carbon dioxide and waste products (as well as excessive proteins through lymphatic drainage).

If this system is impeded in any way, cells, followed by tissues, organs, and entire systems, decrease their level of function. This form of physiological stress then makes the organism vulnerable to disease. To offer an analogy, a good fluid delivery and clearance system is like an open, clean, flowing stream or river. If we block the flow, we have the potential for developing a swamp. Stagnant water allows the buildup of noxious products, and the local environment is completely changed. If we clear the blockage through manual effort, then the stream reestablishes good flow and removes the toxic elements that had begun to build up. The body's own elimination systems can clear toxic waste products produced by cellular damage and allowed to build up by inappropriate tissue tensions, if these tensions are readjusted toward the norm.

Osteopathic manipulation therefore serves as a means not only of decreasing or eliminating pain, but also of adjusting the involved structures. This helps the patient's body to avoid direct noxious stimulus (through compression or excessive stretching) at a macroscopic level, and toxic conditions (through lack of appropriate oxygen/nutrient delivery and to avoid buildup of waste clearance) for cells at a microscopic level. Manipulation is therefore a central issue for osteopathic medicine: though it cannot cure all illness, manipulation is used to help the body function at an optimal level, enhancing its ability to heal itself. The body is capable of amazing feats of self-recovery and may do it more quickly and thoroughly if assisted.

Manipulation, like all forms of medical treatment, has limitations. It is possible that the body's functional levels have been so negatively altered that the use of manipulation alone will not enhance the body's self-adjusting systems enough for it to regain good health (or perhaps to do so within the acceptable time parameters) without the additional assistance of medication or surgery. It may also be necessary to integrate direct psychosocial intervention to affect recovery.

We use medicines and surgery to effect changes in two circumstances: when we feel that preventive measures or manipulation alone will not be able to accomplish our total goal of health (e.g., use of insulin in a type I diabetic, or narcotics in a terminal cancer patient), or when speed is of the essence and our judgment is that it would be dangerous to the patient to simply be manipulated and wait for the body's self-healing responses (e.g., use of antibiotics in overwhelming infection).

Osteopathic physicians who do not use manipulation, but treat patients in a holistic manner, are ignoring a main premise of osteopathic philosophy: assisting the body to eliminate structural impediments that diminish normal physiological function and the body's self-healing capabilities.

LEVELS OF IMPLEMENTATION OF OSTEOPATHIC PHILOSOPHY

There have been conspicuous differences in the evolution of Still's ideas in the United States, and other parts of the world. In the United States, there is a vast spectrum of application of osteopathic principles in the practice of medicine by DOs. Internationally, the application of this philosophy has been different from the United States and involves two levels of training.

In the United States, DOs have always been physicians. Current practitioners implement the osteopathic medical philosophy at various levels along a continuum of medical care. Initially, all osteopathic physicians believed in the efficacy of manipulation to affect the physiology of the body in a positive way. In fact, this has been the hallmark of the osteopathic profession, and Still's development of osteopathic structural diagnosis and treatment was the original reason for the osteopathic profession's existence.

At one end of the continuum, we find the practitioner who practices the pure classic form of osteopathy, using either manipulation or surgery but no medications whatsoever. This type of practitioner is a historical footnote in the development of osteopathic practice in America, and the author knows of no such practitioners at this time. Some physicians accept the importance of manipulation for treatment of pain, but do not see it as having any value in visceral problems. A very few who use manipulation also integrate the homeopathic approach into their practice of medicine.

A small number of osteopathic physicians have chosen to specialize in neuromusculoskeletal medicine, also giving treatment for medical cases in conjunction with treatment by surgical or internal medicine specialists. Some of these practitioners use a minimum of medications, preferring to refer patients who need more intensive medical or surgical care to physicians who likewise specialize in those forms of medical care, including family practice doctors.

Even amongst manipulative specialists, some apply osteopathic techniques in a reductionistic manner, for example, treating only the neck if there is neck pain. This of course negates the osteopathic concept of wholeness, and implies that the physician has not understood that an area of pain may be an area of compensation for a primary problem, rather than being the location of the problem. The physician is neglecting the many muscle and connective tissue connections between the thoracic region and the neck, as well as the sympathetic chain ganglia in the neck that help set the tone for the cervical musculature. While such an approach often works, it frequently is insufficient.

There is an old story that A.T. Still was treating a patient who asked, "Why are you treating me in that area when I have pain down here?" In response, Still related a story of a cat whose tail was rocked over by a rocking chair. The cat experienced pain in the tail, but the shriek of pain came from the other end. This story has been preserved in osteopathic lore as an example of why osteopathic physicians may treat a region of the body that the patient is unaware has problems. The patient has presented with complaints of areas that are dysfunctional in a compensatory fashion, but give the patient pain. It is important to address the primary problem, not just annoying symptoms.

The majority of osteopathic physicians practice in primary care specialties. There is a great range in the amount of OMT that these physicians use with their patients. Others who believe in its efficacy but feel they do not have time to use it with patients may use OMT to treat a friend or relative and will refer patients who need manipulation to physicians who specialize in its use.

Remarkably, there are a number of DOs who have no belief in the efficacy of OMT in clinical application. Some never accepted the osteopathic philosophy nor intended to use OMT, but attended an osteopathic medical college because it was an available pathway to an unrestricted medical license. A subset of these physicians believe that the laying on of hands is, however, valuable to evoke the mind/body or placebo effect. There are also physicians who do not want to be confused with chiropractors and feel that manual therapeutics are best left to physical therapists.

Whether or not they use OMT, virtually all American osteopathic physicians share a profound respect for the body's ability to heal and approach the patient in a holistic manner, viewing the patient as a fellow human being in a unique psychosocial milieu.

The international evolution of osteopathy has been equally complex. After leaving the Chicago College of Osteopathic Medicine (now CCOM at Midwestern University of Health Sciences), J. Martin Littlejohn, a native of the United Kingdom, returned to the U.K. and founded an osteopathic profession in which the practitioners did not use surgery or medicine, and never evolved into a profession with an unlimited medical license.[12] Although these individuals are generally excellent at treating musculoskeletal problems with the use of manipulation, they are currently trying to address their lack of medical acumen in differential diagnosis and do not have the opportunity to prescribe medicine or to perform or assist at surgery or childbirth.

Opinions on this form of evolution vary. American DOs are aware of the dangers in having an expert in manipulation who is not well trained in differential medical diagnosis. Pain might not be recognized as a serious underlying treatable medical or surgical condition, and appropriate treatment may be delayed until it is too late to obtain a favorable outcome. When all that one has is a hammer, too often every problem begins to look like a nail.

International nonmedical osteopathic practitioners, however, would be quick to point out that many American DOs who have an excellent knowledge of medical diagnosis and treatment lack sufficient manipulative skills to effectively treat a patient with a problem where manipulation is clearly indicated.

The British government has recognized the value of including nonphysician osteopathic practitioners in the national health care system. They are generally perceived as specialists in musculoskeletal pain and adjunctive treatment. They are sometimes consulted if the patient has vague complaints and continuing physician efforts do not produce an organic diagnosis. Management of medical conditions is left to the physician. Generally, the public easily identifies this profession and respects the practitioners.

The British Commonwealth spread the nonphysician practice of osteopathic philosophy and manipulation through many countries, and it has been copied in still other European nations. Although these practitioners are called DOs, their degree is Diploma in Osteopathy, rather than the American degree, Doctor of Osteopathic Medicine (formerly Doctor of Osteopathy). The level of training varies. Schools in certain countries have a 4- or 5-year fulltime program; others have a series of weekend courses over several years for physical therapists who wish to become osteopaths.

There is another tier of international osteopathic education, where MD equivalents from various countries have taken postgraduate training in osteopathic diagnosis and manipulation. These practitioners do have an unlimited medical license, and although sometimes lacking in the full knowledge of osteopathic philosophy, in general are similar to American DOs. Many of these physicians integrate osteopathic care into general practice, rehabilitation medicine, sports medicine, rheumatology or neurology, or focus on the conservative treatment of musculoskeletal conditions as well as pre- and postoperative care. France is one country where such training exists. Complicating the picture, French MDs have the legal right to practice osteopathy, whereas those who hold the Diploma in Osteopathy in France do not, but are widely tolerated.

SUMMARY

Osteopathic philosophy is a system of logic for medical diagnosis and care, with rich roots extending back to Greek medicine and beyond. Developed as a system of thought by Andrew Taylor Still, MD, a pioneer physician in Kansas and Missouri, the basic tenets were elaborated by Still in his writings and adopted by the American School of Osteopathy (now Kirksville College of Osteopathic Medicine) as "Our Platform."

The development of additional scientific medicine aided in the evolution of classic osteopathic philosophy to its current form, contemporary osteopathic medical philosophy. The work of Irvin Korr, PhD, a medical physiologist, further elaborated and explained osteopathic theory, including an expanded focus on preventive care and healthful practices.

Osteopathic philosophy uses a holistic approach to begin the analysis of the patient, continuing with a reductionistic approach to focus on aspects of anatomical and physiological dysfunction. One goal of this system of logic is to bear in mind at all steps in the process of diagnosis and treatment that it is a fellow human being with whom we work, even as we zoom in on the smallest microscopic details of the process. No cell or system in the body is seen as acting in isolation, and the importance of structure and function at each level is always kept in mind. Central to this philosophy is a tremendous respect for the innate capacity of the human being to heal, and the physician attempts to work *with* the patient's physiological and psychological processes to obtain an optimal level of homeostasis and function.

Osteopathic manipulative treatment (OMT), the hallmark of osteopathic treatment as developed by Still, is used in patient care, whether alone or in conjunction with medicines and surgery, as appropriate. OMT is recognized as having beneficial effects not only in the treatment of pain, but also to decrease physiological stress and assist the body's self-healing mechanisms.

The application of contemporary osteopathic medical philosophy varies from country to country. There are vast differences not only in its application in the United States and internationally, but also among practitioners in the United States, where osteopathy originated as a distinctive American philosophy and system of medical care.

References

1. American Osteopathic Association: *Yearbook and Directory of Osteopathic Physicians,* Chicago, 1998, AOA.
2. Duffy J: *The healers: a history of American medicine,* Philadelphia, 1979, McGraw-Hill.
3. Educational Council on Osteopathic Principles: *Core curriculum for osteopathic education,* Chicago, 1988, Chicago College of Osteopathic Medicine.
4. Gleick J: *Chaos,* New York, 1987, Viking Penguin.
5. Holmes OW: *Medical essays, 1842-1882,* Boston, 1892, Houghton Mifflin.
6. Korr IM, Ogilvie CD: Health orientation in medical education, United States: the Texas College of Osteopathic Medicine, *Prev Med* 10:710-718, 1981.
7. Northup GW: *Osteopathic medicine: an American reformation,* ed 2, Chicago, 1966, American Osteopathic Association.
8. Singer C, Underwood EA: *A short history of medicine,* ed 2, New York, 1962, Oxford University Press.
9. Still AT: *Autobiography of Andrew T. Still,* Kirksville, Mo, 1897, Author.
10. Still AT: *Osteopathy, research, and practice,* Kirksville, MO, 1910, Author.
11. Still AT: *The philosophy and mechanical principles of osteopathy,* Kirksville, Mo, 1902, Author.
12. Trowbridge C: *Andrew Taylor Still,* Kirksville, Mo, 1991, Thomas Jefferson University Press.
13. Webster GV: Sage sayings of Still. In *Year Book of the AOA,* Los Angeles, 1935, Wetzel Publishing.

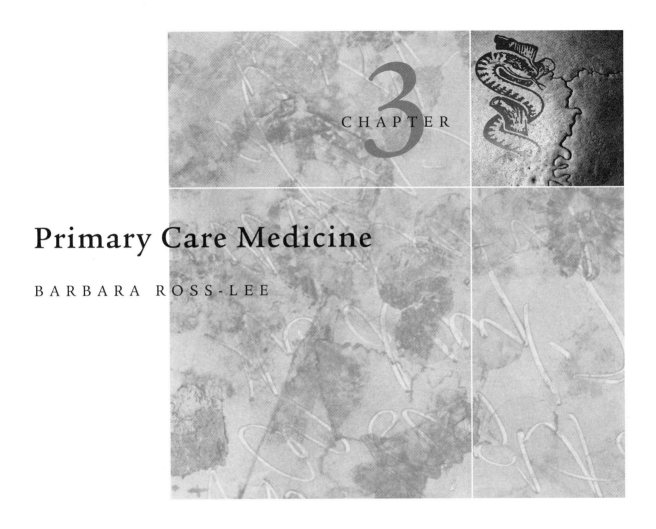

CHAPTER

3

Primary Care Medicine

BARBARA ROSS-LEE

Primary care is the provision of integrated, accessible health care services by clinicians who are accountable for addressing a large majority of personal health care needs, developing a sustained partnership with patients, and practicing in the context of family and community.[8]

Committee on the Future of Primary Care, Institute of Medicine,
Primary Care: America's Health in a New Era

As health care moves into the twenty-first century, the pace of change in the medical professions promises to escalate. Throughout the past decade, the health care industry has witnessed the evolution of managed care and its proliferation in the service delivery sector. Concurrently, managed care's ascendance has increased the value placed upon primary care practitioners and generalist practice. Over the past 70 years, numerous health policy analysts, government agencies, and private foundations and trusts have all recommended the support of primary care medicine and suggested a move away from costly tertiary-care, hospital-based, specialized medicine. Managed care's unprecedented rise as a market force, because of its perceived cost effectiveness, focus on disease prevention and health promotion, and potential to increase access, is serving as a powerful ally to primary care advocates. Under its auspices, the preponderance of health care needs is more efficiently served in ambulatory settings, with a greater portion of health care delivered by generalists.

The emphasis on primary care in the evolving health care environment argues for the reevaluation and reorganization of:

- Medical education—curriculum and methodology
- Medical practice—care settings and practitioner type
- Entire health care infrastructure—integrated delivery systems and interdisciplinary team care

Similarly, the emergence and recognition of nonphysician clinicians (NPCs) as qualified primary care providers ensures a future redefinition of the current concept of *primary care* and promises to challenge the traditional province of osteopathic primary care physicians. The increased presence of NPCs, along with other primary care–specific marketplace trends, guarantees dramatic change in the locus and focus of health care delivery, demands a renewed focus on interdisciplinary care, and signals a need for comprehensive reformation of the medical education process. The call for reform of medical education, as well as medical practice, to accommodate a "managed" care system's need for appropriately trained primary care practitioners is the latest and most effective force in the ongoing 70-year dialogue promoting primary care.

At this juncture in the history of health care in the United States, several options present themselves to the osteopathic medical profession. The direction that the profession chooses to follow at this point in time will likely determine its future status among the health care professions and its future role in a changed and changing system. The current confluence of the osteopathic medical tradition and the nation's primary care agenda indicates that the profession is well positioned to partner with the forces currently driving change in the health care market. Emerging health care systems increasingly require highly trained and skilled primary care practitioners and, if the osteopathic medical profession continues to exhibit its particular proficiency at producing primary care physicians, an analysis of these forces may suggest an appropriate and effective direction for the entire profession. Thus, in order to make sound and well-reasoned choices about the future of the osteopathic medical profession, it is important to review history, assess current strengths, and identify future resource and organizational needs. At the same time, it is imperative to review the history of generalism in the osteopathic medical profession and to trace the path of primary care medicine in this country.

EVOLUTION OF THE PRIMARY CARE/SPECIALTY MEDICINE DIALOGUE

From colonial times through to the latter part of the nineteenth century, the practice of medicine in the United States focused mainly upon curative medicine—the diagnosis and treatment of acute conditions. Physicians throughout this period received medical training primarily through apprenticeships and preceptorships, and then followed mentors into a crude form of general medical practice. These physicians, whether well trained or not, confronted the gamut of maladies and illnesses. Their practices truly represented generalist and essential care for the populace, but the care received often lacked the continuity expected of today's primary care generalists.

Following the end of the Civil War in 1865, physician education shifted to a more formalized institutional training process. The establishment of a greater number of endowed universities toward the end of the 1800s served to increase the number of "educated" physicians, and began to ease medicine out of the trade/apprenticeship stratum and into a more professional occupation status. At the turn of the century, 160 medical schools graduated 5214 and enrolled 25,171 students.[26] The development of a more rigorously defined curriculum in medical education did much to mitigate the purely curative nature of medical practice.

Osteopathic medical practice, separately established as *osteopathy* in the latter part of the nineteenth century, advanced a new and original science of treating illness and disease. Although the exact moment of the formulation of this new science cannot be known, the pivotal ideas seem to have been fully grasped by A. T. Still, MD, in 1874.[5] Dr. Still lost all faith in the efficacy of drug medication in 1864, when the application of drug therapies failed to check the advance of spinal meningitis in two of his own children and in another adopted child.[5] Following this episode, Dr. Still rejected the practice of orthodox medicine and set out to define an entirely new system by which to treat illness and disease. Dr. Still's new science established a new health profession that abandoned the early curative focus of medicine and promoted a "scientific" basis for care focusing on health rather than disease. The orthodox medical science community did not fully comprehend or understand the concepts of the new science.

The principle advanced by Dr. Still, that form and function within the human organism are inextricably linked, along with a broad holistic philosophy, underpins the osteopathic medical profession. Although crudely stated for contemporary medicine, this principle and philosophy arguably resulted in the first true "generalist" theory of practice. In attempting to achieve balance in the whole of the human body and by striving to create and maintain health in the individual, osteopathic physicians appear as the first representation of an articulated philosophy of primary care.

The arrival of the twentieth century witnessed a growing concern for the quality of medical care and, more directly, the quality of medical education. This concern led the American Medical Association (AMA) to engage the Carnegie Foundation for the Advancement of Teaching to sponsor Abraham Flexner's study of the 139 allopathic and 8 osteopathic medical schools operating in the United States, and the 8 medical schools in Canada. Flexner (Figure 3-1) reported an industry-wide lack of minimum educational standards among all schools, and cited specific problems of low entrance standards, poor science laboratory instruction, lack of clinical facilities for bedside training, and inadequate instructional staff. Although many of the individual schools decried the haste with which Flexner "evaluated" their institutions, the *Journal of the American Medical Association* applauded the report and stipulated that the medical profession was long-overcrowded with ill-trained "physicians."[26]

This official denunciation of many providers in that period's practice environment by the AMA, bolstered by evidence in the Flexner report, essentially targeted the "alternative" and "cultist" forms of medical education and was consistent with orthodox medicine's historical desire to squelch or absorb competing practitioners. Even though Flexner predicted and urged that the physician's function become more social and preventive (rather than individual and curative)—

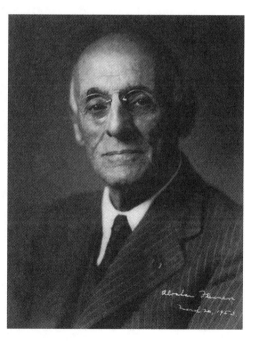

Figure 3-1 Abraham Flexner, a nonphysician commissioned by the Carnegie Foundation to survey medical schools during 1909 to 1910. His study led to the reformation of medical education in the United States. (Courtesy National Library of Medicine, Bethesda, Md.)

essentially calling for a more continuous and primary physician role in patient care—the specific recommendations to the medical schools outlined in his report were inconsistent with this advice and served to neutralize those primary care aspects. Similarly, although he proposed a more social and preventive role for physicians, he did not emphasize population medicine or public health in his curricular endorsements.

The Flexner report, although historically regarded as a watershed in medical education, reinforced many changes already taking place in medical education. The closing of weak schools, the merging of marginal institutions, the hastening of improvements in laboratory and clinical instruction, and the growing trend for schools to align themselves with colleges and universities all began in the decades before Flexner. These previously advanced infrastructure-centered changes, when coupled with his specific recommendations to the medical schools, combined to divert the course of medicine and medical education away from primary care. Flexner believed "that the basic medical sciences should be taught without regard to their medical applications or the student's career goals, and that research, 'untrammeled by near reference to practical ends,' should play a major role in the medical school."[26] Because of his overriding certitude in the scientific method, his report impelled medical educators to emphasize research and academic education rather than professional training, paving the way for the unimpeded growth of medical specialties.

Although Flexner gave great thought to the curricular content of the medical education process he recommended to the schools, he appears to have given scant attention to the scope of the national need with respect to the medical education endeavor. He seems to have had a rather tenuous grasp of national physician workforce needs. Flexner proposed that only 30 4-year schools, enrolling 300 students each, were needed for the entire nation in 1910; this proposal would have reduced the number of graduates by more than 50%, from 4442 to 2000 per year.[14] At this rate of reduction, Flexner's proposal would have added just two physicians per 100,000 people in 1910—the national population stood at just 91 million with 146 physicians per 100,000—and less per year as the population increased.[28]

Flexner's conclusion that none of the eight osteopathic schools was in a position to provide the training that osteopathy required further distanced the profession from orthodox medicine. Labeled a cult practice by allopathic physicians, the osteopathic practitioners were denied access to hospitals controlled and approved by the AMA. Further, under the "standardization of hospitals" plan inaugurated by the American College of Surgeons in 1918 and supported by the AMA, any hospital seeking approval through these two organizations was *required* to prohibit DOs from holding admitting or staff privileges.[16] The lack of privileges in AMA-controlled hospitals, as well as a meager number of osteopathic hospitals and institutions in the early days of this century, confined osteopathic physicians to an almost exclusive role as generalist practitioners.

Inadvertently, Flexner's report—his specific recommendations and his inattention to certain aspects of the educational venture—helped to create a condition of intense physician need at the basic primary level. Although his description of the physician's function urged a more primary care–based role, his educational specifications and shortsightedness compelled the move toward specialization. By championing the academic research archetype, he knowingly promoted the creation of an infrastructure supporting the establishment of medical specialties and the pursuit of medical research and, at the same time, unwittingly encouraged divergent forces in medical education (basic science vs. clinical instruction) and medical practice (specialization vs. generalism). Figures 3-2 and 3-3 compare the effect that both the Flexner report and the development of specialty-based medicine had on the entire (combined) physician population and on the osteopathic medical profession, specifically, over time.

Not surprisingly, only 7 years after the dissemination of Flexner's report, specialty certification—in ophthalmology and otolaryngology—emerged in the United States. By 1997, 80 years later, the Association of American Medical Colleges (AAMC) Data Book listed 161 medical specialties (including subspecialties). The rise in specialty practice in the immediate post-Flexner era, the reduced number of

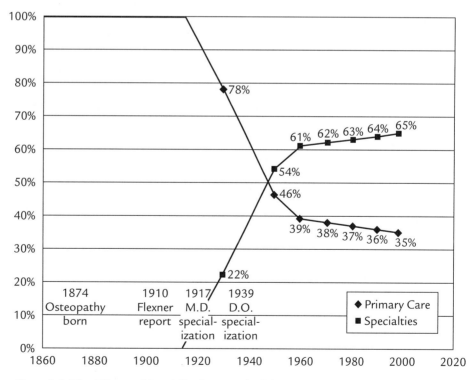

Figure 3-2 The Effects of Specialization on Physician Practice. (Data from Ernst RJ, Yett DE: *Physician location and specialty choice,* 1985, Ann Arbor, MI, Health Administration Press.)

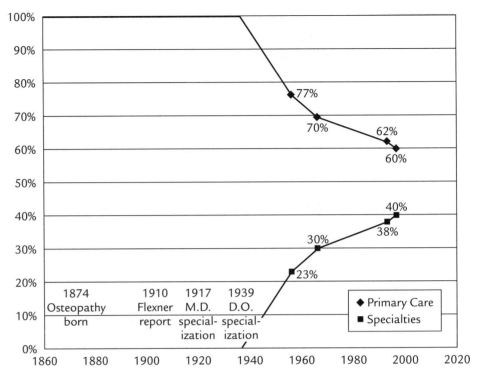

Figure 3-3 The Effects of Specialization on Osteopathic Physician Practice. (Data from AOA Office of Physician Biographical Records and Josiah Macy, Jr. Foundation, Sirica CM, ed: *Osteopathic medicine: past, present, and future,* 1996, Chicago, IL.)

medical school graduates owing to the decrease in the number of medical colleges, and the lack of realistic workforce needs projections produced a sharp decline in the number of physicians available to care for the sick. The number of physicians per capita decreased substantially from 157 physicians per 100,000 persons in 1900 to 125 per 100,000 in 1930.[28] The AMA was widely blamed by physicians and laymen alike for creating this situation.[26] Rural areas of the country suffered the greatest decline in physician representation, since specialists tended to settle in urban areas. The physician-to-population ratio remained at an inappropriate level until the second half of the twentieth century.

Having been effectively barred from the sizable hospitals operated or controlled by the AMA, and having consultations with or referrals to MD specialists deemed unethical by the AMA as well, osteopathic physicians had no choice but to create a parallel organizational infrastructure to pursue a separate professional status.

After an aggressive effort to establish internships in the wake of new licensure requirements spearheaded by the AMA, the AOA proceeded to expand its educational capacity into specialty disciplines. In 1939, in response to a perceived need for standardization of both postdoctoral education and the regulations for certi-fication in the various specialty fields, the Advisory Board for Osteopathic Spe-cialists was founded to address requirements resulting from the growth of spe-cialization in the osteopathic profession. The growth of specialists and subspecialists began as a necessary response to imposed isolation by the allopathic profession but, in contradistinction to allopathic specialization, osteopathic spe-cialization grew out of the generalist tradition. Osteopathic specialists came from the ranks of the osteopathic general practitioners. As late as the 1950s, nearly all practicing osteopathic specialists, including those establishing the various spe-cialty residency training programs, were DOs who had voluntarily limited their practices, studied independently, and trained with any specialist who would al-low them the privilege.

In spite of the forces initiated by Flexner, which served to distance physicians from patients, the patient-physician relationship shifted from sporadic and episodic care to a pattern of continuing association as evidenced by the popular-ization of the periodic health examination in the 1920s. Periodic health exami-nations became an accepted part of medical care and established the belief that both healthy and ill patients should consult the physician regularly. Physicians, as a result, started accepting responsibility for a specific patient base, began to keep longitudinal medical records on patients, and began to develop long-term rela-tionships with patients and families. However, even as more and more physicians accepted this new general care method of practice, an increasing number of physi-cians continued to opt for specialization. These specializing physicians elected to remove themselves from first-contact care, choosing instead to provide consulta-tive care by referral only.

As osteopathic medicine gained professional and organizational strength, a number of significant events began to alter the AMA's stand on osteopathic med-icine. The Joint Commission on Accreditation of Hospitals revised its policy in 1960 to permit a hospital having an "osteopath" or "osteopaths" on its staff to apply for accreditation provided that it was listed with the American Hospital As-sociation (AHA).[26] The AHA likewise amended its hospital listing requirements to include hospitals having doctors of osteopathy on their staff—if evidence of "regular" care was submitted—effectively ending years of imposed isolation. How-ever, it was not until the Report of the Board of Trustees on Osteopathy, in De-cember 1968, that the AMA revised its position on osteopathic medicine, encour-aging county and state medical societies to "accept qualified osteopaths" as members.[25]

The AMA's change of position, although viewed as a success in the osteopathic medical profession's desire to achieve equality between it and orthodox medicine, created new hurdles in maintaining a separate and distinct profession. Just 25 years after the change, as of 1993, 63% of DO residents in training have opted to train—and been accepted—in allopathic residencies, an amazing turn of events considering the historical biases held by allopathic physicians against osteopathic physicians. This reversal is consistent, of course, with the shift toward generalist care and the allopathic programs' emerging desire to produce primary care physicians and to fill their burgeoning primary care positions funded by Medicare graduate medical dollars. In 1993, after prior failed attempts, the American Academy of Family Physicians, a national allopathic organization, finally endorsed full membership for osteopathic physicians.[25]

Despite the historic official denunciation of the osteopathic medical profession, a few allopathic and osteopathic physicians did develop relationships, both personal and professional. Allopathic specialty programs first trained osteopathic physicians as favors to friends or colleagues. Osteopathic physicians would be trained in these programs but would not be counted among the allopathic residents or given staff privileges after completion of the training. This sporadic allopathic training of DO graduates accelerated because of several specific changes in the allopathic profession's position toward osteopathic physicians; these changes had a direct impact on the training opportunities afforded osteopathic medical graduates. One of the events facilitating the flow of osteopathic physicians to allopathic residencies was the directive from the Secretary of Defense, Robert McNamara, in 1966, instructing the army, navy, and air force to accept qualified DOs as officers in the medical corps. As DOs entered the armed services, the only manner in which they could receive formal postdoctoral training while on duty was in federal hospital programs, which were not accredited through the AOA. After leaving the military, these allopathically trained DOs were welcomed in allopathic hospitals and sometimes headed up training programs where they practiced. In turn, these osteopathically influenced programs tended to consider more applications from DOs.

A review of select aspects of the osteopathic profession's turbulent history reveals the adversity that the profession has had to endure to survive and thrive. Because of the allopathic-imposed isolation, the profession had to pursue specialization out of necessity. But, because of the nature of the osteopathic philosophy and holistic core of its educational model, the profession has maintained a distinctive generalist focus. Figure 3-4 shows that the osteopathic medical profession has maintained a strong and consistent primary care base (family practice, internal medicine, and pediatrics) near 60% throughout the last decade. However, the entire medical profession has experienced a profound reduction in the number of physicians practicing in the generalist specialties and in primary care during the past 65 years (from near 80% to only 30%), chiefly because of the allopathic medical profession's headlong pursuit of specialization.[25] By far, the majority of osteopathic physicians engage in family practice (46.5%)[20], adjudged by the recent Institutes of Medicine (IOM) panel as the most appropriate setting for the majority of primary health care needs.[8] Even as osteopathic medical graduates pursue graduate training in allopathic medical programs, they tend to fill excess slots in the primary care specialties created in response to Medicare funding and left va-

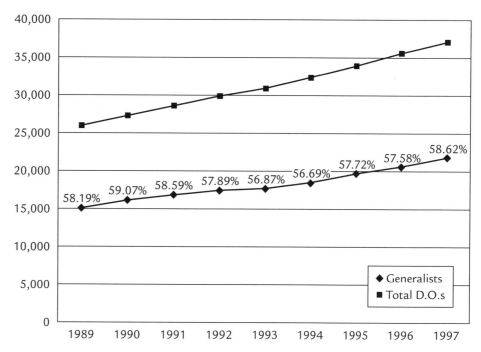

Figure 3-4 Osteopathic Primary Care Physicians—circa 1990s. (Includes family general medicine, general internal medicine, and general pediatrics.) (Data from AOA Office of Physician Biographical Records, Yearly Data Books 1989-1997, Chicago.)

cant by allopathic medical graduates. The 1996 AMA Annual Survey of GME Programs reported 3288 osteopathic graduates in allopathic programs (61% of the 5429 DO residents that year) and gave the breakdown of specialties with the highest osteopathic representation (Table 3-1).

The Pew Foundation, the Robert Wood Johnson Foundation, the Macy Foundation, the Council on Graduate Medical Education (COGME), and the AAMC have all made specific recommendations for change strategies, which if adopted by medical schools, will facilitate the production of more primary care physicians. The specific strategies proposed by these organizations essentially reproduce the "osteopathic" educational model:

- An admissions policy that preferentially accepts students who profess an interest in primary care
- An admissions and recruitment strategy that accepts the nontraditional student who more frequently selects a primary care career path
- An admissions policy that seeks to add minority representation
- Significant primary care representation on admissions committees
- Primary care included in the school or college's mission statement
- Establishment of departments of family medicine in parity with other traditional clinical departments

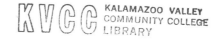

TABLE 3-1

Specialty Choice of Osteopathic Medical School Graduates in Allopathic GME Programs[2]

Choice	Number	Percentage
Family practice	852	26
Internal medicine	695	21
Pediatrics	239	7
Psychiatry	183	5.5
Emergency	150	4.6
Ob/Gyn	149	4.5
Physical medicine & rehabilitation	113	3.4
Other	907	28
Total	3288	100

From JAMA 278:775-776, 1997.

- Required curriculum courses and clerkships in primary care disciplines
- Increased training in nonhospital settings
- Increased emphasis on community-based training with community-based practitioners
- Tenure and promotion criteria that emphasize teaching
- Significant integration of biopsychosocial and prevention into the predoctoral curriculum
- Early and continuous clinical contact for predoctoral students
- Changes in the core curriculum
- Creation of community-centered partnerships

Throughout the history of the osteopathic medical profession, the core philosophies have focused upon a holistic approach to medical care and have established an unrivaled tradition of primary care practice. Although osteopathic physicians necessarily have had to venture into the arena of specialization and subspecialization, the osteopathic specialties nonetheless issue from a strong generalist foundation. In 1994, the 32,209 active osteopathic physicians represented just 4.5% of the 716,623 active physicians in this country, and yet they constituted more than 20% of the family/general practitioners in the country.[20] The osteopathic medical profession's strong 60:40 ratio of generalists-to-specialists supports a higher family practice and primary care presence. As Figure 3-5 shows, the generalist-to-specialist ratio for the allopathic profession has dipped below 35:65 for the last two decades and accounts for the profession's relatively poor performance in supporting the nation's call for primary care physicians.[20] Similarly, osteopathic physicians exhibit a 59:41 ratio of practice in nonmetropolitan areas to metropolitan areas, while allopathic physicians post an 11:89 ratio respectively.[4]

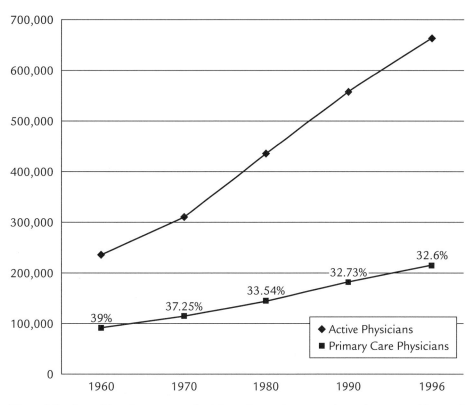

Figure 3-5 Allopathic Primary Care Physicians. (Counting general practice, general internal medicine, and general pediatrics.) (Data from Physician Characteristics and Distribution in the United States, AMA, 1997, Chicago.)

Clearly, osteopathic physicians, despite their small numbers, have positioned themselves to address the concerns of physician maldistribution and the need for increased primary care to a greater degree than have their allopathic counterparts.

CALL FOR THE REFORM OF MEDICAL EDUCATION AND PRACTICE

As the generalist and specialist paths diverged at an increasing rate, several adverse consequences, as a result of increased specialization and suppressed generalist care, revealed themselves. The expanded research activities among the scientific community had resulted in great advances in the treatment of illness and disease, but the general population had not always benefited from this progress. Often, medical care cost more than many patients could afford, and access to care was limited in many parts of the country. The trend toward specialty care and away from generalist care, firmly established in the first quarter of the twentieth century, created concerns in the mid-1920s about the adequacy of care and the distribution of physicians throughout the country. These concerns have persisted over time and questions of cost, quality, and access to care have been addressed repeatedly in numerous studies. Invariably, the reports reiterated and emphasized a need for increased primary care as a basis for improving the health status of the population but, until recently, few of the reports focused specifically on population medicine or public health as a means to that end. The reports also consistently acknowledge the proliferation of specialty practice and its negative impact on access to general patient care. Through expanded research activities, specialists succeeded in adding new modalities, medical devices, and medications to the physician's armamentarium, with the potential to increase the general health status of the population. However, the increased specialization in the physician workforce decreased the general population's ability to gain access to these innovations in care.

To explore the unsatisfactory delivery of basic care in the United States, the Committee on the Costs of Medical Care (CCMC), a private group established on May 17, 1927, undertook the task of the first comprehensive study of health care in this country. In the CCMC final report, adopted October 31, 1932, the Committee reported that the inexcusable level of preventable physical pain and mental anguish, needless death, economic inefficiency, and social waste within the medical profession was largely unnecessary. Within the section of the report titled "An Ultimate Objective", the Committee urged that in an ideal setting, "each patient would be primarily under the charge of the family practitioner . . . [and] . . . would look to his physician for guidance and counsel on health matters and ordinarily would receive attention from specialists only when referred to them by his physician."[7] In the report's recommendations, the Committee suggested that the needs of the people called for three to five times as many well-trained general practitioners as specialists.[7]

Another study, undertaken by the Commission on Medical Education in the mid-1920s, also published its final report in 1932 concerning the general nature of medical education in America. The Commission's survey of recent medical school graduates of the period reported the students' view that an inordinate amount of the schools' clinical education was delivered by specialists, with an overemphasis both on the problems of research and on those diseases most commonly seen by specialists; student consensus indicated that insufficient attention was given to the basic needs of most patients.[12]

However, the expansion of medical specialties brought with it a concomitant increase in the level of medical research and technological invention and development. From 1850 to 1899, the efforts of American scientists accounted for just 13% of the compiled list of medical discoveries, behind the French with 14% and the Germans with 46%. From 1900 to 1926, American scientists jumped into the lead with 33% of all discoveries.[26] The arrival of World War II sparked the quest to promote wartime medical innovations in the government's comprehensive effort to address medical problems associated with war. The government gave 450 contracts to universities and 150 contracts to private research institutes, hospitals, and others—at a cost of $15 million—to pursue the development of wartime technologies.[15] Following the end of the war, the increased momentum of research in the medical fields carried research efforts to an unprecedented level. Financial support from the National Institutes of Health brought Flexner's vision of a specialized, research-dominated, university-centered medical education model to fruition. The research grants naturally emphasized a specialization of effort, since most of the proposed research called for highly technical and specialized expertise. The great sums of money that researchers could bring to colleges and universities set in motion a vicious cycle where dollars meant respect, prestige, and power. Since the specialties dominated the research fields, more and more allopathic physicians turned to the specialties, which, in turn, led to the immediate depletion of the generalist ranks—a situation that persists to this day.

As a means of providing distinctive skills in primary care for allopathic generalist physicians and as an avenue for gaining a small portion of available research dollars, the American Academy of General Practice was organized in 1947; residencies in general practice were established the following year in 1948. This effort to gain an equal degree of prestige and respect among fellow allopathic physicians did not immediately gain a level of recognition comparable to board certification in the established specialties. In 1959 the American Board of General Practice was incorporated, but interest in the new board waned until it obtained acknowledgment from the American Academy of General Practice in 1967 and the Liaison Committee for Specialty Boards in 1969. Renamed the American Academy of Family Practice (AAFP) in 1969, to reflect its specialty status, it became the first American specialty board to institute mandatory recertification requirements. In 1972 the American Osteopathic Board of General Practice came into existence; it has since changed its name to the American Osteopathic Board of "Family" Physicians.

During this same period, Kerr White and colleagues contributed to the concept and study of primary care in a 1961 article titled "The Ecology of Medical Care." White and associates articulated a concept defining the chief role of medical "care" research as being concerned with "the social, psychologic [sic], cultural, economic, informational, administrative and organizational factors that inhibit and facilitate access to and delivery of the best contemporary healthcare to individuals and communities."[30] By investigating the process by which a person perceived a disturbance in their health and then initiated the quest for care, the authors defined a "primary unit of illness" and consequently enunciated a concept of primary and continuous care.

From 1960 to 1980 the concept of primary care was continuously refined in several key reports:

- 1965 - AAMC - *Planning for Medical Progress Through Education* submitted by Lowell T. Coggeshall, MD—better known as the Coggeshall Report—examined the trend of increased medical specialization within the context of rising demands for basic health care among the populace. The report urged the development of a "team" approach to patient care and called for a means to produce more family physicians. The report also argued that medical education should be viewed as a continuum and that the concept of medicine as a single discipline should be replaced by the concept of "health professions" working in concert to maintain and increase the health of society as well as the individual.[6]

- 1966 - AMA - *The report of the Citizens Commission on Graduate Medical Education,* chaired by John S. Millis, PhD—known as the Millis Commission Report—defined the primary care physician as the primary medical resource and counselor to an individual or a family.[10]

- 1973 - Joel J. Alpert, MD, and Evan Charney, MD, in conjunction with the U.S. Department of Health, Education, and Welfare - *The Education of Physicians for Primary Care* sought to critically review the educational programs designed to prepare physicians to practice primary care. Drs. Alpert and Charney identified the three fundamental characteristics of the primary care physician as (1) establishing first-contact medicine, (2) assuming longitudinal responsibility for the patient regardless of the presence or absence of disease, and (3) serving as the "integrationist"/coordinator-of-care for the patient. They suggested a reallocation of financial support to increase the production of primary care physicians and urged some limitation on the availability of subspecialty careers.[1]

- 1976 - The Josiah Macy, Jr. Foundation - *Physicians for the Future* examined the short supply of physicians in many localities across the country. The report revealed severe physician shortages in rural areas and inner cities and found that the nation's increased demand for medical services, combined with changing patterns of medical practice, had resulted in a loss of access to physicians. The report also found that the bulk of private physicians, mainly specialists, lacked the ability to fulfill patients' need for comprehensive primary care.[21]

- 1978 - Institutes of Medicine (IOM) - *Manpower Policy for Primary Health Care* defined essential primary care as "accessible, comprehensive, coordinated, and continual care provided by accountable providers of health services (as distinguished from public, environmental, and occupational health services), where initial professional attention is paid to current or potential health problems."[19] The IOM report urged an increase in the number of primary care practitioners (as well as fair reimbursement for their services), and stressed that an adequate percentage of physicians must be trained in the primary care specialties and be proficient in the full range of primary care practice skills.

- 1978 - World Health Organization (WHO) - *Alma-Ata 1978: Primary Health Care* documented the proceedings of the International Conference on Primary Health Care held in Alma-Ata, USSR, and issued a declaration expanding the definition of primary care. The Alma-Ata Declaration articulated a highly symbolic goal of "Health for All by the Year 2000," and stated that "Primary Health Care is essential health care made universally accessible to individuals and families in the community by means acceptable to them, through their full participation and at a cost that the community and country can afford. It forms an integral part both of the country's health system of which it is the nucleus and of the overall social and economic development of the community."[31]

In 1976, the Graduate Medical Education National Advisory Committee (GMENAC) undertook the first detailed specialty-by-specialty study of the U.S. physician manpower needs using a consistent and acceptable methodology. Since previous work in this area was fragmented, partial, and often outdated, the Committee had to devise the report's methodology from the ground up. The GMENAC report, issued in 1980, warned of explosive growth in the output from American medical schools and predicted a surplus of 70,000 physicians in 1990 and 145,000 in 2000. The GMENAC report, recognizing the overproduction of specialists, recommended that medical school graduates in the 1980s be encouraged to enter training in the generalist fields.[29]

In 1983, Drs. Joseph H. Abramson and Sidney L. Kark, in their pioneering study on communities and the community connection with health practitioners, advanced the concept of Community Oriented Primary Care (COPC). Drs. Abramson and Kark defined COPC as a "strategy whereby elements of primary health care and of community medicine are systematically developed and brought together in a coordinated practice"[18] using hospital services, public health practice, and primary health care in the community. The doctors recognized the Alma-Ata Declaration as a source for their focus on the integration of clinical primary care and community medicine.

The close of the 1980s brought a realization that evolving health care systems, moving rapidly to managed care, demanded a substantial increase in the number and proficiency of primary care practitioners. Comprehensive reform of the health care system became a major platform in the 1992 presidential election, but proved to be an unattainable goal of the Clinton administration. Political infighting, as well as the enormity of the task, doomed all attempts at a national solution to the country's health care problems. The national debate, however, did spur attempts to influence the production of primary care physicians and resulted in a plethora of reports on the subject; several of those reports are summarized below.

- 1992 - The Council on Graduate Medical Education (COGME), Third Report- *Improving Access to Health Care Through Physician Workforce Reform* enunciated the "Health Care Crisis" and defined the triad of concerns—inadequate ACCESS to care, poor and/or unequal health status within the population (QUALITY), and the high COST of health care. In the report's first finding, COGME declared that the Nation has too few generalists and too many specialists. In recognizing the critical need for primary medical care in any health care system, the report listed the following elements of primary care:
  - First contact care for persons with undifferentiated health concerns
  - Person-centered, comprehensive care that is not organ or problem specific
  - An orientation toward longitudinal care
  - Responsibility for coordinating other health services as needed[9]
- 1993 - The Pew Health Professions Commission (Pew) - *Health Professions Education for the Future: Schools in Service to the Nation.* The report's fourth recommendation called for schools to employ a *generalist-interdisciplinary orientation,* citing a widespread consensus that the nation's health care needs require a system that is properly balanced between specialized and primary care.[24]
- 1995 - Pew - *Critical Challenges Revitalizing the Health Professions for the Twenty-First Century* stressed the need for an emphasis on primary care within health professions education and acknowledged that emerging health care systems would be integrated through the delivery of primary care. The report advised that all health practitioners, *generalists and specialists,* be able to understand the values and functions of coordinated, comprehensive, and continuous care and direct their practices to support such goals.[23]
- 1996 - IOM - *Primary Care: America's Health in a New Era* established a new definition of primary care as "the provision of integrated, accessible health care services by clinicians who are accountable for addressing a large majority of personal health care needs, developing a sustained partnership with patients, and practicing in the context of family and community." An important, but unpublished indication of the committee members was that of the generalist specialties, family practice provides the most appropriate setting for treating the majority of health care needs—based on frequency and incidence.[8]
- 1999 - National Fund for Medical Education (NFME) - *Primary Care Action: First Things First for Our Health Future,* a white paper from the NFME, laid out a "vision for a radically different approach to primary care, one that focuses on the needs of publics and consumers served, rather than the immediate interests of the professions themselves." *Primary Care Action* seeks

"to advance the health of individuals, their families, and communities by strengthening, evolving and advancing primary care principles, practice, and leadership in the United States." The core values of the initiative include "universal access to health care, creative redeployment of health care resources to achieve new efficiencies, effective management of health care to produce the highest levels of quality, and creation of a 'health commons' to promote the public's health."[22]

For 70 years, the specialist and generalist paths have diverged—the generalist-to-specialist ratio has steadily declined over the years. Members of the public—both professional and lay—have repeatedly decried this trend and the health care industry's inability to produce a necessary level of primary care physicians to meet society's needs. Issues of cost, access, and quality in health care appear repeatedly throughout the succession of reports over the years and remain critical factors in health care as the industry moves into the twentieth century. Although the majority of the recommendations listed in the reports have gone largely unheeded, piecemeal interventions have attempted to right the skewed physician representation and distribution in the country.

Policy decisions at the federal and state levels have contributed to the confusion over the kind of physicians the nation should train. Agencies like the Health Resources and Services Administration have supported primary care initiatives through grants and study commissions, and the National Health Services Corps and Indian Health Service Corps have used scholarships and loan programs to train and place physicians in underserved areas of the country. These programs required service from the physicians they trained, but not necessarily primary care specialization. Only recently did the Bureau of Health Professions change the Health Professions Student Loan program under Title IV to the Primary Care Loan program and require commitment to primary care practice. They also added this requirement to the Exceptional Financial Need Scholarship and Financial Aid for Disadvantaged Health Professions Students programs.

However, other agencies, such as the Health Care Financing Administration (HCFA), have historically instituted policies that have promoted the training of specialists through the creation of skewed financial incentives, such as the incentives that guide graduate medical education funding through the Medicare program. Even though the original objective of HCFA was to increase the number and quality of physicians, the payment system for graduate medical education inadvertently left the primary care agenda behind. By paying hospitals' direct and indirect costs for residency programs, HCFA has supported specialty training in the large tertiary care hospitals of the academic health centers. Since the establishment of Medicare in 1965, the number of residents in the system has ballooned to 103,661 in 1994/1995; only 35% have opted for primary care training. In 1994/1995, the allopathic medical profession filled 25,796 of the available residency slots with international medical graduates (IMGs)—more than 50% of these IMGs filled vacant primary care discipline slots—in order to meet the demand created by the skewed financial incentives. In addition, policy support for research and development of medical technology, largely in relation to the specialty disciplines, has risen steadily with the budget for the National Institutes of Health. Only the fledgling Agency for Healthcare Research and Quality has made specific attempts to carry out research in support of knowledge in primary care medicine.

Even the Hill-Burton Act of 1946, enacted to encourage the construction of hospitals and to increase patient access to health care, had unintended consequences where the osteopathic profession was concerned. By funding the osteopathic hospital ventures around the country, the Act made the training of large numbers of specialists in a hospital setting a reality for the osteopathic profession. Records documenting the emergence of osteopathic specialists are scarce, but as training programs increased and subsidization of medical schools by the federal government expanded in the 1960s, the generalist-to-specialist ratio in the osteopathic profession began to decline. Several surviving copies of the yearly *A Statistical Study of the Osteopathic Profession* from the late 1950s to the late 1960s provided data for Figure 3-6, and illustrate that by the mid- to late-1960s the osteopathic generalist-to-specialist ratio had dropped to 70:30.

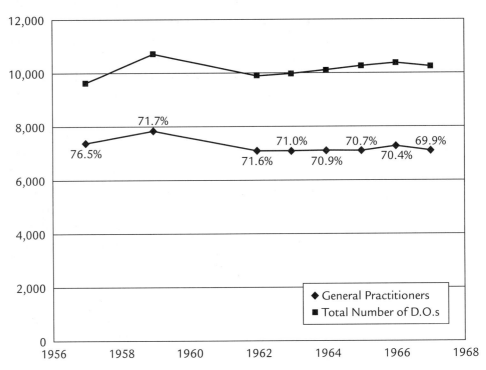

Figure 3-6 Osteopathic General Practitioners—circa 1960s. (Includes general practice [no specialty attention] and physicians limited to manipulative therapy.) (Data from A Statistical Study of the Osteopathic Profession AOA, 1957-1967, Chicago.)

At the state level, Medicaid funding for graduate medical education has followed the pattern set by the Medicare program and has also compromised the production of primary care practitioners. Although many states established new medical schools in the 1970s, with a mission of training primary care physicians, only a few have delivered on that mission (mainly the osteopathic medical schools). The failure of comprehensive health care reform at the national level in the early 1990s prompted the development of market-driven strategies to address the need for improvement in the efficiency of the health care industry. By focusing on managed care's emphasis on, and demand for, primary care practitioners, these strategies have begun to redress the imbalance of generalists to specialists.

Even as the most recent policy strategies have attempted to increase the number of primary care practitioners emerging from the education pipeline, the skewed financial incentives remain in place. A recent study of physician compensation conducted by the Medical Group Management Association (MGMA) gives cause for renewed concern. The *Physician Compensation and Production Survey,* based on 1996 compensation information from 30,812 physicians reported that growth in specialty physicians' compensation outpaced those of primary care physicians, a reversal of a 5-year trend. According to the survey, primary care physicians earned an average $135,217—an annual growth rate of 1.42% for 1996, whereas specialists earned an average $221,544—growing at 2.58%.[11] The *Medical Economics Continuing Survey,* also relying on 1996 figures, confirmed the MGMA report and stated that, in most cases, physicians overall were unable to keep up with the rate of inflation.[17]

PRIMARY CARE–CHALLENGES AND OPPORTUNITIES FROM TODAY'S EVOLVING MARKETPLACE

In the last decade of the twentieth century, the demand and value placed upon primary care practitioners increased dramatically; primary care experienced a true renaissance. In the early 1990s, the growth of managed care organizations precipitated a rise in the demand for primary care physicians to act as gatekeepers in order to manage the perceived over-use of specialty services—this "gatekeeping" model has since been waning in actual practice. In the 1990s, the health care field also witnessed a marked increase in both the number of medical school graduates choosing primary care specialties and in the salaries paid to these providers, after decades of salary stagnation in relation to the more highly rewarded specialty fields. Finally, the numerous recommendations from think-tanks, agencies, trusts and foundations, and various policy makers, as well as the numerous reform measures brought at the state and federal levels throughout the 1990s, have predominantly focused on the necessity of expanding the ranks of the nation's primary care workforce.[27] However, in the absence of a clear consensus in the health care industry to decrease the overall production of physicians, the call for increased numbers of primary care providers confound a perceived oversupply in the total provider pool.

Although the trends in these areas bode well for the future of "primary care" in the new millennium, several emerging trends may, in fact, signal distinct challenges to the primary care "physician" in the immediate future. Some of these trends include (1) managed care's move away from the gatekeeper model; (2) innovations in information technology that promote patient education, access to care, and continuity of care; and (3) rapid growth of nonphysician clinicians and expansion in their scopes of practice providing an enhanced opportunity for the delivery of both disease care and health care.[27]

This last trend, the growth of nonphysician clinicians, the expansion of their historical scopes of practice, and the increasing degree to which they have begun to take over the primary responsibility for first-contact care, poses a direct challenge to the established province of osteopathic primary care physicians unless proactively engaged. Osteopathic primary care physicians, in large numbers, have traditionally served in rural and urban underserved regions, increasing the access to health care services for vulnerable and underserved populations. Nonphysician clinicians (NPCs)—nurse practitioners (NPs), physician assistants (PAs), and certified nurse midwives (CNMs)—have advanced claims that they too serve these vulnerable populations, can manage up to 80% of the patient's primary health care needs, and can do so at a greatly reduced cost. These claims, bolstered by potential savings in time and resources needed to train the NPCs, make them attractive as alternative providers in the nation's quest for an increased primary care workforce.

PRIMARY CARE AND THE FUTURE OF OSTEOPATHIC MEDICAL EDUCATION AND PRACTICE

As the osteopathic medical profession enters the twentieth century, demands of the marketplace and the evolving health care delivery and finance system continue to drive changes in medical education, medical practice, health workforce composition, and in the entire health care infrastructure. In the midst of this continuous and overlapping process of change, the demand for primary care-focused medical education, primary care–driven business organization, and primary care services occupies a place of preeminence in strategy debates. Osteopathic medicine's success in producing generalist physicians, with their potential for increasing access to underserved and vulnerable populations, creates a strong position for the profession. Ironically, a portion of the credit for this successful positioning must be shared with the allopathic medical profession. The osteopathic medical profession stands as a product of imposed isolation, and much of the profession's development as a parallel medical profession with parallel status came as a direct response to outside pressures and discrimination by the allopathic profession.

Having met the challenges of a minority profession and having achieved practice parity with allopathic counterparts, the osteopathic medical profession is much freer to choose the direction that it will follow into the next century. The historical isolation suffered by the osteopathic profession largely extended to the denial of opportunities to access the same resources, which the allopathic profession ultimately over-used. Thus, the profession did not experience the impact of the same skewed incentives toward specialization that have created the cost-prohibitive allopathic tertiary care system. At this critical point in health care evolution, amidst demands for an increased primary care presence, the osteopathic educational model and profession can serve as an example as the allopathic profession attempts to respond to external changes and extricate itself from the burdensome and often inefficient system that it has created. As the health care industry collectively grapples with the certainty of future reforms, necessitating changes in medical education and medical education financing, medical practice (locus and focus), and the basic health care infrastructure, the relatively small size of the osteopathic profession allows it to institute change rapidly.

At this point in time, the osteopathic medical profession is uniquely situated to take a strong and active part in leading the process of addressing the nation's need for primary care physicians. To control its own destiny in the changing marketplace, the profession should focus on its innate strengths, particularly its dominance in family practice. Armed with its successful primary care educational model, the profession has an opportunity to join the forces of change in negotiating health policy, which supports a medical education program consistent with the nation's evolving health care delivery and medical practice needs. The osteopathic medical profession has already made significant strides to enhance and reorganize its medical education system, strengthening its ability to produce better-prepared physicians for future practice. Most osteopathic schools have the commitment to primary care in their mission statement. Thus, assuming a leadership stance in the production of primary care physicians allows the osteopathic medical profession to maintain a separate professional status in the health care arena. By taking on a leadership posture, the osteopathic profession can embark on a path away from merely occupying a parallel existence and toward a truly distinctive presence, in relation to the allopathic profession. Innovative changes to the osteopathic educational infrastructure represent the first step on the path.

The consortium approach to graduate medical education (GME) has been embraced by the profession through its new accreditation process for osteopathic graduate medical training, creating a vertically integrated medical infrastructure and the potential for a coordinated medical education continuum linking undergraduate and graduate medical education. In July 1995, the American Osteopathic Association Board of Trustees passed a controversial new regulation for the accreditation of osteopathic GME by establishing the Osteopathic Postdoctoral Training Institutes (OPTI) system. The OPTI system sets the standards for the minimum number of residency programs, as well as numbers of interns and residents to be trained by the OPTI, and requires college affiliation for all GME programs.

By adopting a leadership posture at this unique moment in the evolution of the health care delivery system, distinctiveness may be preserved and enhanced. The holistic philosophy of the osteopathic profession, the focus upon disease prevention and health promotion as well as the socioeconomic, psychosocial, and sociocultural aspects of the individual's need for care, provides an appropriate foundation for a primary care education. The osteopathic philosophy also emphasizes the relationship between structure and function in the human body. Thus, the practice of manual medicine adds a distinctive and valuable component to the osteopathic armamentarium, which will become increasingly important in providing both cost-effective care and chronic care. The profession, particularly the primary care portion, is endowed through its educational system with distinctive/unique skills that enhance palpatory diagnosis, enable cost-effective manipulative therapeutic interventions, and integrate the healing touch in patient care. Research in health status indicators, outcomes of manual medicine techniques, curricular reform, and the dissemination of new knowledge will continually renew and validate the osteopathic educational model.

The dedication to primary care, prevalent throughout the osteopathic profession makes change and leadership in primary care an attainable goal. However, to be strong in primary care education, the profession must be community-based. Accreditation in the allopathic profession, through the Liaison Committee for Medical Education, is based on a hospital's number of beds and has supported the inefficient tertiary care model. The osteopathic medial profession, not saddled with this type of hospital-dependent infrastructure, possesses the potential, through its army of community volunteer faculty, to become truly community-based.

> Prodded by purchasers seeking lower costs, greater efficiency, and better outcomes in primary health care, the hospital environment of just 10 years ago has undergone major changes. Those changes are forcing medical educators to peer outside the hospital walls into the community to equip physicians-in-training with the right mix of technical and patient skills they will need when they begin practicing.[13]

Market forces emphasizing primary care and calling for a decrease in specific specialty production, as well as the merging of hospitals into broader systems of care—not just allopathic or osteopathic—have already mandated much of the course for the future. Building upon the osteopathic profession's strength and occupying a lead position in the production of distinctively trained primary care physicians carves out an important niche for the profession. Capitalizing on that strength will connect the future of osteopathic medicine with its philosophical core and guide successful primary care policy initiatives in partnership with the powerful forces driving change in the marketplace.

References

1. Alpert JJ, Charney E: *The education of physicians for primary care,* Washington, DC, 1973, US Depart Health, Education, and Welfare.
2. American Medical Association: Appendix II, graduate medical education, *JAMA* 278:775-76, 1997.
3. American Medical Association: *1995-96 Physician characteristics and distribution in the United States,* Chicago, 1996, American Medical Association.
4. American Osteopathic Association: *Yearbook and directory of osteopathic physicians, 1996,* Chicago, 1996, American Osteopathic Association.
5. Booth R: *History of osteopathy and twentieth-century medical practice,* Cincinnati, 1905, The Caxton Press.
6. Coggeshall LT: *Planning for medical progress through education,* Evanston, Ill, 1965, Association of American Medical Colleges.
7. Committee on the Costs of Medical Care: *Medical care for the American people; the final report,* Chicago, 1932, University of Chicago Press.
8. Committee on the Future of Primary Care, Institutes of Medicine, Donaldson MS, Lohr KN, and Vanselow NA, eds: *Primary care: America's health in a new era,* Washington, DC, 1996, National Academy Press.
9. Council of Graduate Medical Education: *Improving access to health care through physician workforce reforms: direction for the 21st century,* Third report, Rockville, Md, 1992, US Depart Health and Human Services.
10. Council on Medical Education and Hospitals: *The graduate education of physicians: report of the Citizens' Commission on Graduate Medical Education,* Chicago, 1966, American Medical Association.
11. Dunevitz B: Specialty physicians' compensation outpaces those of primary care, *Medical Group Management Update* 36:1-2, 1997.
12. *Final report of the Commission on Medical Education,* New York, 1932, Office of the Director of Study, 1932.
13. Firshein J: Coming into the community:building a new model for US medical education. In Josiah Macy, Jr Foundation, Sirica CM, ed: *Current challenges to M.D.'s and D.O.'s,* New York, 1996, Josiah Macy, Jr Foundation.
14. Flexner A: *Medical education in the United States and Canada: a report to the Carnegie Foundation for the Advancement of Teaching,* Boston, 1910, The Merrymount Press.
15. Foote SB: *Managing the medical arms race: public policy and medical device innovation,* Berkeley, 1992, University of California Press.
16. Gevitz N: *The D.O.'s: osteopathic medicine in America,* Baltimore, 1982, Johns Hopkins University Press.
17. Goldberg JH: Are boom times over for primary care? *Medical Economics,* 74:217-29, 1997.
18. Institutes of Medicine, Connor E, Mullan F, eds: *Community oriented primary care: New Directions for Health Services Delivery,* Washington, DC, 1983, National Academy Press.
19. Institutes of Medicine: *Manpower policy for primary health care,* Washington, DC, 1978, National Academy Press.
20. Josiah Macy, Jr Foundation, Sirica CM, ed: *Osteopathic medicine: past, present, and future,* New York, 1996, Josiah Macy, Jr Foundation.

21. Macy Commission: *Physicians for the future: report of the Macy Commission,* New York, 1976 Josiah Macy, Jr Foundation.
22. National Fund for Medical Education: *Primary care action: first things first for our health future,* San Francisco, 1999, University of California, San Francisco Center for Health Professions.
23. Pew Health Professions Commission: *Critical challenges revitalizing the health professions for the twenty-first century,* San Francisco, 1995, Pew Health Professions Commission.
24. Pew Health Professions Commission: *Health professions education for the future: schools in service to the nation,* San Francisco, 1993, Pew Health Professions Commission.
25. Ross-Lee B, Kiss LE, and Weiser MA: The outlook for osteopathic medical specialists within a reformed healthcare system, *J Am Osteopathic Assoc* 96:558-67, 1996.
26. Rothstein WG: *American medical schools and the practice of medicine,* New York, 1987, Oxford University Press.
27. Sagin T: Are primary care physicians riding the crest or entering the trough? *New Medicine* 2:9-14, 1998.
28. United States Bureau of the Census: *Historical statistics of the United States: colonial times to 1970,* Part 1,Washington, DC, 1970, US Depart Commerce.
29. United States Graduate Medical Education National Advisory Commission: *Report of the Graduate Medical Education National Advisory Commission,* Washington, DC, 1980, US Depart Health & Human Services.
30. White KL, Williams F, and Greenberg BG: The ecology of medical care, *N Eng J Med* :265:885-893, 1961.
31. World Health Organization: *Alma-Ata 1978: primary health care,* New York, 1978, World Health Organization.

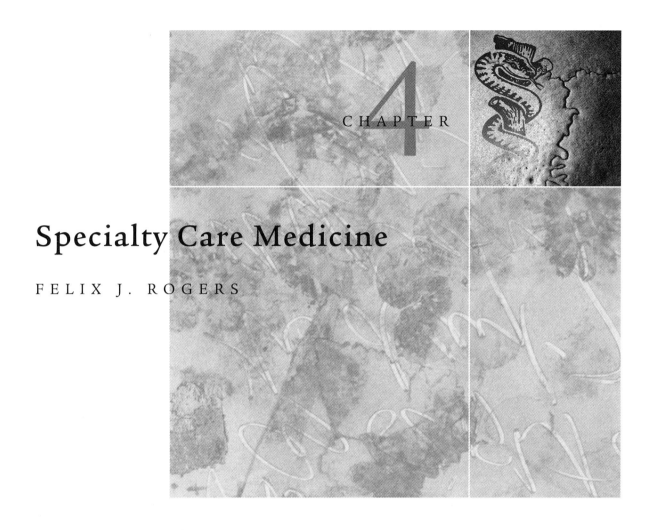

CHAPTER

4

Specialty Care Medicine

FELIX J. ROGERS

The object of life is not to be on the side of the majority, but to escape finding oneself in the ranks of the insane . . .

MARCUS AURELIUS

At first glance, some people find osteopathic specialty care to be antithetical to the osteopathic concept and the practice of osteopathic medicine as they have come to understand it. After all, osteopathic physicians have established a special place in American health care. They are noted for their role as primary care physicians and their health care work in small towns and in underserved parts of the country, especially rural areas. Also, historically, osteopathic hospitals have served as small, general community hospitals. These developments are not a necessary outcome of osteopathic principles but, instead, may be a consequence of external factors related to medical licensure, access to postgraduate training, dominance of the allopathic academic and health care system, and other issues that are described in earlier chapters of this book. The tenets of osteopathic medicine are as applicable to medical practice in specialty areas as they are in family practice. In fact, the perspective of the physician giving specialty care may bring into focus aspects of comprehensive patient care that will enhance the ability of the primary care physician to approach the patient from a holistic perspective.

Although the traditional strength of osteopathic medicine has been in primary care medicine, osteopathic physicians now provide health care within all specialties and most subspecialties of medicine and surgery. Each specialty college establishes standards for residency training and certification. The American Osteopathic Association (AOA) Council on Postdoctoral Training oversees each of the specialty programs. The graduate of a specialty residency is first and foremost an osteopathic physician. The training incorporates the knowledge base and clinical skills necessary to provide primary care to patients from adolescents to geriatrics, along with the social and academic skills also needed to effectively serve this entire population. In addition, the unique concepts and skills of osteopathic medicine are emphasized and blended throughout the training years.

Specialty training takes place in osteopathic hospitals, in allopathic institutions, and in hospitals with a combined staff. Approximately 65% of all DOs who are in residency training programs complete their study in an allopathic institution. Osteopathic physicians successfully compete for spots in some of the top postgraduate training programs in the country. After completion of the residency training programs, osteopathic physicians may sit for certification examination by the osteopathic board. In some instances, certification by an osteopathic board carries with it automatic recognition by the corresponding allopathic specialty college. For example, a DO certified in cardiology by the American College of Osteopathic Internists is automatically eligible to become a Fellow of the American College of Cardiology.

BRIEF HISTORY OF OSTEOPATHIC SPECIALTIES

The following history of osteopathic specialties is taken from a concise summary published by the AOA Department of Educational Affairs: *Handbook of the Bureau of Osteopathic Specialists*. It describes the regulatory component of specialties within the AOA.

The Bureau of Osteopathic Specialists (hereinafter also referred to as the "Bureau") was organized in 1939 as the Advisory Board for Osteopathic Specialists to meet the needs resulting from the growth of specialization in the osteopathic profession. It was thought at that time that there should be standardization of postdoctoral education and regulations for certification in the various specialties or fields of practice. Therefore, the Board of Trustees of the American

Osteopathic Association, through its agency, the Advisory Board for Osteopathic Specialists, became the certifying body.

In the early development of the various specialty groups in the osteopathic profession, the certifying boards not only served as examining bodies for their candidates, but also were responsible for the development of the various types of postdoctoral educational programs, including residencies, preceptorships, and subspecialty residencies (formerly known as assistantships or fellowships) (Table 4-1).

Until 1948, the Advisory Board was the clearing house and the final agency for recommending directly to the AOA Board of Trustees regarding specialty ed-

TABLE 4-1

Certifying Boards in Specialties or Fields of Practice Within Osteopathic Medicine

Certifying boards	Year established
American Osteopathic Board of Radiology	1939
American Osteopathic Board of Surgery	1940
American Osteopathic Boards of Ophthalmology and Otolaryngology—Head and Neck Surgery (formerly the American Osteopathic Board of Ophthalmology and Otorhinolaryngology, 1940-1996)	1940
American Osteopathic Board of Pediatrics	1940
American Osteopathic Board of Proctology	1941
American Osteopathic Board of Neurology and Psychiatry	1941
American Osteopathic Board of Internal Medicine	1942
American Osteopathic Board of Obstetrics and Gynecology	1942
American Osteopathic Board of Pathology	1943
American Osteopathic Board of Dermatology	1945
American Osteopathic Board of Rehabilitation Medicine	1954
American Osteopathic Board of Anesthesiology (formerly under the Board of Surgery)	1956
American Osteopathic Board of Family Physicians (formerly the American Osteopathic Board of General Practice, 1972-1993)	1972
American Osteopathic Board of Nuclear Medicine	1974
American Osteopathic Board of Special Proficiency in Osteopathic Manipulative Medicine (formerly the American Osteopathic Board of the Fellowship of the American Academy of Osteopathy, 1977-1990)	1977
American Osteopathic Board of Orthopedic Surgery (formerly under the Board of Surgery)	1978
American Osteopathic Board of Emergency Medicine	1980
American Osteopathic Board of Preventive Medicine (formerly the American Osteopathic Board of Public Health and Preventive Medicine, 1982-1983)	1982

*The American Osteopathic Academy of Sports Medicine was established in 1989 to award a certificate of competence.

ucation and certification of candidates. In December 1948, the Committee on Accreditation of Postgraduate Training was established to evaluate training programs in specialties other than for hospital residencies. The Bureau of Hospitals had largely taken over the approval of residencies in the specialty fields existing at that time by 1943. In many instances, the Bureau of Hospitals actually set up the training regulations for residencies.

As the specialty organizations developed, the various specialty affiliates, beginning with the American College of Osteopathic Surgeons, became responsible for the development of educational formats in their specialty fields. At the present time, these specialty affiliates are responsible for educational programs through their evaluating committees, and the certifying boards are responsible for the examination of candidates for certification.

In January 1968, the Committee on Postdoctoral Training (COPT) replaced the Bureau of Hospitals for purposes of approval of postdoctoral training. In 1993, the Committee was renamed the Council on Postdoctoral Training (COPT). In March 1989, the AOA Board of Trustees provided the Advisory Board with the authority to review the appropriate documents of any AOA specialty affiliate proposing a certificate of competence or an earned fellowship. In July 1991, the Board of Trustees changed the terminology to "certificate of special recognition," and in July 1992, to "certificate of added qualifications." In February 1994, the term was modified to "certification of added qualifications." Thus, certificates of special recognition or competence are no longer issued.

In 1993 the Board of Trustees changed the name of this body from the Advisory Board to the "Bureau."

ROLE OF OSTEOPATHIC SPECIALISTS IN MEDICAL CARE

How do osteopathic specialists contribute to the practice of osteopathic medicine and, in turn, participate in the general reformation of medicine in the United States? This chapter explores the answers to this in an assessment of (1) the use of osteopathic manipulative therapy as a tool to implement the osteopathic philosophy, (2) the incorporation of osteopathic tenets into specialty practice, (3) the role of specialists in expanding osteopathic concepts, and (4) the role of osteopathic specialists in health care delivery systems.

Osteopathic Manipulative Treatment and Specialty Care

Since its inception, osteopathic medicine has been a minority profession with a specific philosophical emphasis. Although it has been pressured to prove itself in the scientific arena, most of the energies of the profession in its early years were expended on battles for full licensure and equal medical practice rights. A distinctive feature of the osteopathic profession is that it has endeavored to establish guiding principles to represent a philosophical and scientific basis for health care. Although the basic tenets of the profession[19] are broad, individuals within and beyond the osteopathic profession have typically chosen an emphasis on osteopathic manipulative treatment (OMT) as a defining element of osteopathic medicine. It is crucial to remember that OMT is a tool for applying a philosophy, and not the philosophy itself. It is more proper to state that the osteopathic profession has traditionally recognized a central role of the neuromusculoskeletal system in disease and in health maintenance.

Historically, palpatory diagnosis and OMT played a major role in osteopathic medicine. Interestingly, little is known about the manipulative therapy techniques actually used by Andrew Taylor Still and his first generation of students. A considerable period of time elapsed before any techniques were recorded. In the middle of the twentieth century, the vast majority of osteopathic physicians practiced a type of manipulation characterized as high-velocity, low-amplitude, or "thrust" manipulation. Over the past 50 years, a wide variety of manipulative techniques have been developed, including myofascial release and counterstrain, and manipulation has been supplemented with mechanical devices such as percussion hammers. The remarkable evolution of OMT in the past 50 years has been matched by other approaches to the neuromusculoskeletal system including exercise, yoga, acupuncture, and other physical modalities. Because so many other health care providers have learned manipulative techniques from osteopathic physicians, none of these interventions are exclusively within the domain of the osteopathic profession. The key feature is the philosophical orientation behind the application of these methods of health care, with an emphasis on the central role of the neuromusculoskeletal system.

In practice, osteopathic medicine is a method of health care delivery implemented by an individual physician's approach to patient-physician relationships. In some cases, the musculoskeletal system is the focus of the patient encounter because it is either the primary expression of disease or because of its integral relationship to health and/or a disease process. In these cases, musculoskeletal palpatory diagnosis and osteopathic manipulative therapy represent issues of such central importance that they are both necessary and sufficient for patient care. For example, for patients with the common problem of low back pain, osteopathic manipulative treatment is applied as a modality of proven efficacy. Palpatory findings are sufficient, and in general, radiological or other diagnostic studies are not needed in patients with uncomplicated cases. There are other clinical disorders within the fields of orthopedic medicine, obstetrics, sports medicine, physiatry, and pain management in which there are clear indications for osteopathic manipulative therapy that allow for the most complete expression of comprehensive patient care management.

Within the specialty fields of medicine, there are specific situations for which the musculoskeletal system is a key component to health or the derangements of a disease process. For example, in the field of neurology, the use of palpatory diagnosis and manipulative treatment has long been an effective part of the management of patients with headache. In obstetrics, the application of OMT during the latter stages of pregnancy and during labor and delivery is well recognized for its clinical effectiveness. Asthma is a clinical condition in which the musculoskeletal system plays a major role in chest wall and ventilatory dynamics; somatic and visceral interactions mediated through the autonomic nervous system provide a rationale for OMT. In the field of cardiology, the application of OMT is much less common than is the widely accepted intervention of cardiac rehabilitation exercise for patients with coronary heart disease and heart failure. However, OMT does have a major place in the evaluation and treatment of patients with noncardiac chest pain. The textbook *Foundations for Osteopathic Medicine*[25] provides a current summary of the application of osteopathic concepts in each of these and other fields.

In other clinical settings, the role of the musculoskeletal system in disease processes is more peripheral, and the use of OMT is adjunctive rather than primary. In many cases, this has happened as a result of the evolution of new diagnostic and treatment modalities. For example, the development of effective antihypertensive agents has moved OMT to an adjunctive role in the treatment of hypertension, in contrast to a legitimate interest in studying the effectiveness of OMT as a primary modality a few decades ago. Similarly, the development of new imaging techniques and other diagnostic modalities has pushed the palpatory diagnostic examination to a position of less prominence. However, these facts do not deny the historical or present importance of palpatory diagnosis and OMT. The goal of osteopathic medicine is not to prove the efficacy of OMT, but instead to provide the best possible care for patients. If a medical innovation proves to be a superior modality, embracing that advance and incorporating it into patient care is the effective means to implement the osteopathic philosophy.

In clinical practice, the use of OMT by osteopathic specialists has undergone considerable evolution and often varies from one specialty to another. A close look at the evolution of procedures related to the field of surgery illustrates this point. Before the establishment of the American College of Osteopathic Surgeons (ACOS) in 1927, osteopathic physicians were almost exclusively primary care physicians whose practices concentrated on manipulative treatment. Although they might have had skills in suturing wounds or performing minor surgical procedures, formal training programs for such skills did not exist at that time. The ACOS was established because the founding members wanted to incorporate osteopathic concepts into the practice of surgery. Until about 25 years ago, many of the individuals who entered a general surgery residency program first honed their skills in osteopathic principles and practice by going into primary care medicine, before their residency in surgery. Presently, nearly all surgical residents enter a residency directly after their internship.[16]

The basic tenets of osteopathic medicine are comprehensive philosophical principles that should be incorporated into the preoperative evaluation of a patient, intraoperative management, and postoperative care. There was a time in the osteopathic profession when every patient in an osteopathic hospital received OMT as part of routine postoperative care. OMT was often performed by house officers as well as by the surgeon. Treatment was intended to minimize the major postoperative complications of pneumonia, postoperative atelectasis, and postoperative ileus.

Improvements in surgical technique and anesthetic agents, the advent of minimally invasive surgery (e.g., laparoscopic cholecystectomy), and early ambulation have all had a major impact on the reduction of these complications. Partly because of the prevention of these complications, the use of OMT by surgical specialists has decreased dramatically over the past few decades. In some instances, the need for postoperative OMT has been met by a defined service of osteopathic manipulative medicine (OMM) in the hospital. For example, at the Detroit Osteopathic Hospital, OMT was routinely performed by a specialist in OMM for every patient who had open heart surgery. Although patients accepted this procedure favorably and praised its effectiveness, there was no systematic documentation of its efficacy. In addition, no data are available concerning the degree to which primary care physicians subsequently incorporated OMT into a post hospital care plan that also included cardiac rehabilitation exercise, risk factor modification, diet planning, and other lifestyle changes.

This example of the use of OMT in the postoperative open heart surgery patient highlights a controversial issue related to the application of OMT in patient care. Should every osteopathic physician be skilled in OMT and treat their patients with this modality? Although there may not be a definite answer to this question, there are parallel issues in the practice of medicine. There are certain medical problems that are so common that they represent public health concerns of sufficient magnitude that every physician should have basic skills in the recognition and treatment of these disorders, which include hypertension, diabetes, hypercholesterolemia, and basic cancer screening. If a specialist sees a patient in consultation for a separate problem and identifies uncontrolled hypertension or diabetes, multiple factors come into play regarding the need for the specialist to intervene in this problem that is outside of his or her area of specialty. Is the problem so acute that it requires immediate attention? Is the primary care physician already aware of this problem? Has a management plan already been established? Does the patient belong to a managed care entity that requires all evaluation and management to be conducted by the primary care physician unless a referral is made?

These same questions can be asked concerning musculoskeletal problems and the opportunity for the specialist to intervene with appropriate OMT. In most situations, the practice patterns will define what occurs. When well-established referral patterns incorporate frequent and open communication between the specialist and the primary care physician, and when both sets of physicians share common treatment goals, the clinical situations are much more easily resolved. At a minimum, it can be readily established as to which physician will provide OMT for the patient. Several areas of consensus probably exist: (1) every DO should have at least basic skills in osteopathic palpatory diagnosis and OMT, (2) the ideal situation is one in which OMT is integrated into a continuity of care and is used by both specialists and primary care physicians, and (3) the most likely occurrence is that OMT is most commonly employed by the primary care physician or the OMM specialist.

Examples of the skillful integration of OMT into specialty care are well described in several chapters of *Foundations for Osteopathic Medicine*. Shaw and Shaw[18] describe the therapy of sinusitis in a manner that exemplifies the integrated osteopathic approach of a specialist. The discussion begins with the review of the anatomy and physiology of the nose and paranasal sinuses. Next, the pathophysiology of sinusitis is reviewed, with an emphasis on inflammation, structural changes, and the role of the sympathetic nervous system. The diagnostic tests include palpatory testing of the head and neck, paraspinal areas, and Chapman's reflex points, in addition to computed tomographic images of the sinuses. Treatment includes the categories of patient instruction and participation and musculoskeletal, medical, and surgical interventions.

The management of women during pregnancy represents another situation where the specialist or the generalist can take the lead in promoting the use of osteopathic palpatory diagnosis and OMT. Low back pain is one of the most common complaints and complications of pregnancy and has traditionally been accepted as inevitable by women and their physicians. Predisposing factors and mechanisms of low back pain are complex and incompletely defined.[22]

The osteopathic approach to the pregnant patient begins with the first prenatal visit. During the first trimester, musculoskeletal considerations include a palpatory structural examination to identify an abnormality of the somatic system that could affect the outcome of pregnancy, advice concerning exercise, and OMT as appropriate. During the second trimester, complaints related to musculoskeletal changes continue. The next most common musculoskeletal complaint during pregnancy involves the hands and wrists, especially carpal tunnel syndrome (CTS). Whereas it virtually always resolves soon after birth, palliative therapy is indicated for CTS for the more symptomatic patient. Myofascial technique has been shown to be effective for this condition.[20,21] During the third trimester, mechanical and structural changes in the woman become maximal. Osteopathic manipulative treatment can be helpful to mobilize fluid from the extremities to the systemic circulation and to relieve somatic dysfunction.

The approach a neurologist takes in caring for a patient with headache clarifies the difference between osteopathic manipulation and mere manual medicine. Manual medicine can be any form of treatment applied by the hands. The term *osteopathic manipulation* indicates that the physician is implementing the osteopathic philosophy in patient care, including the four basic tenets of osteopathic medicine.[19]

The International Headache Society Classification (IHSC) of headaches (Table 4-2) includes twelve different classifications of headache, and a thirteenth category for headache that cannot be classified. Although OMT may be beneficial in the treatment of headache, it is not good for all types of headache, and the specific manipulative approach taken varies according to the pathophysiology of the headache. Elkiss and Rentz[5] reviewed the use of OMT in migraine, cluster, and tension headache.

OMT may be a valuable part of nonpharmacological therapy for the treatment of migraine headache. In the active phase of migraine, gentle therapy with indirect technique and venous and lymphatic drainage techniques are more likely to be helpful during the attack. Treatment is directed at the lower cervical and upper thoracic vertebrae, associated ribs, and myofascial attachments. There may be musculoskeletal triggers to migraine; OMT can be used in an attempt to modify these triggers. Other nonpharmacological approaches include biofeedback, applications of local heat or cold, massage, accupressure, trigger point therapy, acupressure, traction, or local anesthetic blockade.

Cluster headache is a distinctive vascular syndrome characterized by attacks that occur daily for weeks at a time and then vanish for months or years. They are associated with autonomic vasomotor features and may refer pain to the cervical and upper thoracic paraspinal region, as well as the suprascapular area. OMT is best directed at these areas, the associated soft tissues, and the relevant craniofacial structures.

Tension-type headaches are the most common headache type. They are mild to moderate in severity, pressing or tight in quality, typically bilateral, and usually occipital in location. Treatment starts with elimination of offending situations, such as medication overuse, drug dependency, or depression. Then inquiry for a history of emotional, physical, or sexual abuse is completed. And finally, the physician identifies and eliminates the potential musculoskeletal triggers such as the teeth, jaw, sinuses, and adjacent musculoskeletal and paraspinal structures.

In headache management, the presence of somatic dysfunction should be systematically identified and managed with OMT. Special care needs to be taken with manipulation of the cervical spine because of complications that may occur, although such complications are infrequent. Elkiss and Rentz[5] provide a comprehensive table describing the key features in treatment for 15 types of headache resulting from systemic disease or a primary neurological disorder; for only one of these is OMT indicated. For others it is not helpful or may even be contraindicated.

TABLE 4-2

Headaches Resulting from Systemic Disease or Primary Neurologic Disorder

Disorder	Pathophysiology	Clinical features	Paraclinical features (lab, x-ray, etc.)	Treatment
Glaucoma	Increased intraocular pressure	Dilated pupil, disturbed vision, general headache	Abnormal tonometry	Medication, surgery
Cerebral aneurysm, ruptured or unruptured	Berry aneurysm, hypertension	Explosive headache, nuchal rigidity, abnormal neurologic	Blood in the CSF, abnormal angiogram	Neurosurgery
Temporal arteritis	Inflammation	Throbbing headache, >55 years old, tender temporal artery, blurred vision, jaw claudication	Elevated ESR, positive biopsy for arteritis	Glucocorticoids
Optic neuritis	Inflammation, demyelination	Orbital pain, loss of vision, worse with eye motion, papillitis	Abnormal visual evoked response, abnormal MRI	Glucocorticoids
Dissection of carotid, vertebral arteries	Drugs, trauma	Severe, local pain, tender artery, Horner's syndrome	Angiogram, ultrasound, MRI	Surgery, anticoagulators
Temporomandibular joint syndrome, internal derangement, myofascial	Joint degeneration, muscular imbalance	Pain in jaw, click in joint, locking of joint, pain with lateral or vertical movement, tight muscles	Abnormal MRI	Dental, physical therapy, exercise
Trigeminal neuralgia	Irritation of CN-5, vascular loop, mechanical	Sharp, stabbing pain in trigeminal zone, triggers: wind, eating, chewing	Rarely abnormal MRI	Medication (anticonvulsant) neurosurgery
Herpes zoster trigeminalis cervicalis	Infection	Burning pain hypersensitive rash/vesicles	Virus identification	Antiviral therapy

CSF, cerebrospinal fluid; ESR, erythrocyte sedimentation rate.
From Elkiss ML and Rentz LE: Neurology, in Ward RC, editor: *Foundations for Osteopathic medicine,* 1997, Williams & Wilkins.

Implementation of Osteopathic Tenets

The basic tenets of osteopathic medicine were established by a working group at the Kirksville College of Osteopathy in 1953.[19] The four key principles of osteopathic philosophy are:

1. The body as a unit; a person is a unit of body, mind, and spirit.
2. The body is capable of self-regulation, self-healing, and health maintenance.
3. Structure and function are reciprocally interrelated.

TABLE 4-2

Headaches Resulting from Systemic Disease or Primary Neurologic Disorder—cont'd

Disorder	Pathophysiology	Clinical Features	Paraclinical Features (lab, x-ray, etc.)	Treatment
Meningitis encephalitis	Usually infection bacterial, viral, etc.	Nuchal rigidity acute headache, fever, signs of infection	(+)CSF pleiocy-tosis, low glu-cose, high protein	Antibiotics, corticos-teroids supportive
Sinusitis, facial oteomyelitis	Infection	Nasal obstruction, tender bone, fever	Leukocytosis, abnormal CT/MRI	Antibiotics
Intracranial hypertension from a mass	Traction, dis-placement of painful struc-tures, block of CSF, hydrocephalus	Recent onset, headache, worse at rest, papilledema	Abnormal CT/MRI	Glucocorti-coids, furosem mannitol, neurosurgery
Benign intracranial hypertension	Altered CSF dynamics	Young, female, obesity, hormone fluctuating sight papilledema	Increased CSF pressure, small ventricles, en-larged blind spot	Glucocorti-coids, aceta-zolamide, CSF removal, neurosurgery
Exertional headache, strain, life, cough, exercise, coitus	Posterior fossa mass, Chiari malformation, migraine variant	Abrupt, severe, lasts 15-20 minutes, men > women	CT/MRI	If no mass, pre-ceeds active with NSAIDS
Normal pressure hydrocephalus	Communicating, block in CSF absorption	Ataxia, incontinence, dementia	Hydrocephalus, cisternography	Ventrical shunt, CSF removal
Myofascial pain syndrome	Trauma	Bands, nodules, trigger points, poor sleep		OMT, spray/stretch, needling

4. Rational treatment is based upon an understanding of the basic principles of body unity, self-regulation, and the interrelationship of structure and function.

The perspective of the osteopathic specialist allows the incorporation of these elements into everyday practice. In a world of super specialists in medicine, it is not at all uncommon for a view of the whole patient to be lost because of the frag-mentation of care that occurs as the patient receives technologically advanced and sophisticated care. Often, this has such obvious consequences that the entire med-ical community is shocked to learn of such events. For example, at some of the finest academic health care centers in the country, patients undergo percutaneous transluminal coronary angioplasty as part of the treatment for advanced coronary atherosclerosis, which occurs as the result of the development of obstructive cholesterol plaques within the circulation to the heart. A retrospective study of the charts of these patients indicated that more than 80% of them had been discharged home from the hospital without first having a laboratory test performed to measure their serum cholesterol levels or were discharged without receiving any advice or counseling on the causes of cholesterol build-up or information about how they might prevent future episodes of coronary atherosclerosis.

Profiles of treatments offered for patients with coronary heart disease and heart failure show a tendency to underuse highly effective therapy and to instead provide treatment of dubious or proven negative value. In some cases, this may reflect intense marketing pressures that seem to persuade physicians to think in terms of a limited number of treatment options (Table 4-3). Irrespective of the reason, this tendency to use treatment that is ineffective or harmful is a phenomenon that is now significantly diluted in comparison to the widespread use of harmful or dangerous practices that motivated Andrew Taylor Still to establish osteopathic medicine in the late nineteenth century. One hundred years ago, many treatment methods were directly dangerous or harmful. Today physicians have the advantage of randomized clinical trials and evidence-based consensus statements to guide treatment. Nonetheless, there is an ongoing, continuous need to be vigilant about the use of treatment programs that are effective, as opposed to those that are popular or based on anecdotal experience.

In addition to the four standard osteopathic tenets, there are several widely accepted concepts within the field of osteopathic medicine that include (1) the

TABLE 4-3

Use of Interventions to Reduce Risk of Recurrent Myocardial Infarction or Cardiac Death in Patients with Previous Myocardial Infarction

Treatment	Estimated %, frequency of use	% Risk reduction for recurrent cardiac events
Diet	20	35-55
Exercise	10	45
Smoking cessation	20	50-70
Angiotensin-converting enzyme inhibitor	60	40
Aspirin	70	40
Beta-blocker	40	20
Calcium-channel blocker	50	? none
Cholesterol-lowering drug	30	30-40
Estrogen replacement therapy	20	40-50

Modified from Vogel RA: *Coron Artery Dis* 6:466-471, 1995. Printed with permission from *J Am Osteopathic Assoc* 96:28-30, 1996.

rule of the artery is supreme, (2) somatovisceral and viscerosomatic reflexes are central components of body unity, (3) the neuromusculoskeletal system is the primary machinery of life, and (4) OMT is the primary modality for treatment of the musculoskeletal system. Osteopathic specialists can be helpful in interpreting these concepts in the context of their specialty area. For example, within the field of cardiology, the "rule of the artery is supreme" is now interpreted in terms of the role of endothelial function and is evaluated in the management of patients with acute myocardial infarction in the context of the open artery hypothesis.

At the time Andrew Taylor Still formulated the axiom "the rule of the artery is supreme," arterial vessels were believed to be passive conduits for blood flow. Subsequently, vascular tone was thought to be controlled solely by vascular smooth muscle. A more dynamic view of the behavior of healthy and diseased arteries focuses on endothelial function. The endothelium is a regulatory organ that mediates homeostasis, contractility, cellular proliferation, and inflammatory mechanisms in the vessel wall; it has a major role in the development of atherosclerosis. One hundred years ago, Still was concerned about bony impingement that would affect arterial flow externally. Presently, our view has evolved to assess factors in the interior of the vessel that affect coronary blood flow. As it turns out, the same factors that we consider to be risk factors for the development of coronary heart disease are the factors that impair endothelial function: smoking, hypertension, hyperlipidemia, diabetes mellitus, and atherosclerosis. The chemical substance that causes blood vessels to expand normally when there is a need for increased blood flow is endothelium-derived relaxing factor (EDRF). This has been described as the body's own nitroglycerin,[8] and it might be considered as an example of a medicine that the body produces to promote its own healing, a concept that echoes original statements of A.T. Still.

Discoveries within the specialty areas of medicine have shed new light on the role of viscerosomatic and somatovisceral interrelationships and have made a contribution to original osteopathic thinking. For example, an investigation of angina has given us new insights into the heart as an internal organ responding to painful stimuli. The concept of silent ischemia that has developed over the last two decades has now been balanced by the discovery of the "hypersensitive heart." It is now clear that there is a spectrum of responses to ischemia and that an individual may lie anywhere on that continuum. At one end are the hypersensitive patients that are plagued by incessant symptoms that may just represent simple premature contractions. At the other end are the 25% of patients with myocardial infarction that occurs as a silent or unrecognized event.

The somatic manifestations of myocardial pain have been well studied by osteopathic physicians. Collaborative research between specialists in osteopathic manipulative medicine and cardiologists have demonstrated consistent abnormalities in the paraspinal musculature in patients with angina pectoris and acute myocardial infarction.[1,3,12] Other investigators have examined the anatomic location of anginal pain in relationship to the site of ischemia[4] or the location of myocardial infarction.[13,15] Drawing on a knowledge of viscerosomatic reflexes, specialists have applied interventions such as transcutaneous electrical nerve stimulation or dorsal column stimulation to stimulate the area of the musculoskeletal system that reflects the anginal pain. Somatic stimulation in the areas of perceived pain not only reduces the frequency of angina, but also improves exercise tolerance[6,11] and, in some studies, even increases coronary arterial blood flow.[2]

Expansion of Osteopathic Tenets

Medical specialists can play a leading role in the modern interpretation of osteopathic philosophy. Consider the role of the neuromusculoskeletal system as a central component in the role of health maintenance and in disease. Although palpatory diagnosis and OMT has historically been the primary modality used to assess and treat the musculoskeletal system, a variety of specialty approaches have provided new insight and effective treatment within osteopathic medicine. For example, radiographical procedures that use magnetic resonance imaging (MRI) have shown that there are specific, localized abnormalities in the neck muscles of patients who have chronic headache.[7] This provides substantial evidence for a musculoskeletal component to chronic headache and represents a foundation for further investigation for the application of OMT as part of headache management. MRI is also being used in the study of somatic dysfunction, which was previously called the "the osteopathic lesion."

Interventions to benefit the musculoskeletal system may enhance OMT. For example, flexibility and stretching exercises, aerobic exercises, and strengthening exercises are recommended as adjunctive therapy to osteopathic manipulative treatment.[9] Likewise, Tai Chi and other forms of balancing exercise are recommended in the orthopedic community to help protect against falling and subsequent hip fracture.[17] Cardiac rehabilitation programs incorporate aerobic exercise and strength training exercises to assist patients in their efforts to regain functional status and return to work. Other examples of neuromuscular interventions that build on osteopathic concepts of somatovisceral interaction and the primary role of the musculoskeletal system include transcutaneous electrical nerve stimulation, acupuncture, yoga, bio-feedback, and relaxation techniques. Individuals in the physiatry, rheumatology, and psychiatry specialties may also recommend these.

Osteopathic specialists have joined forces with primary care physicians in making prevention and nutrition key elements of a modern interpretation of osteopathic concepts. The works of A.T. Still and the early practitioners of osteopathic medicine did not emphasize nutrition. Increasingly, a concentration on nutrition counseling, risk factor modification, and preventive medicine has represented a component of the distinctiveness of osteopathic medicine.

HEALTH CARE DELIVERY SYSTEMS

Health care reform has been a subject of national debate throughout the decade of the 1990s. Typically, it has been reduced to the simple concern of decreasing health care expenditures. A more comprehensive view of health care includes the following:

1. Prevention
2. Managing primary care
3. Managing specialty care
4. Managing hospital care
5. Care at the time of terminal illness

Intrinsic to this health care reform is a desire to improve the quality of medical care and to reduce its cost. Increasingly, it appears that managed care may do one or the other, but not both.

Because osteopathic medicine centers on the patient-physician relationship, both the primary care physician and the osteopathic specialist have a major stake in this national dialog on health care reform. The present environment puts financial imperatives over philosophical principles and threatens to jeopardize the patient-physician relationship. Osteopathic physicians need to be vigilant in insisting that their professional obligation must remain that of being advocates for patients' well being and not that of being employees of a health maintenance organization with duties to stockholders as opposed to patients.

One trend in the approach to the patient is to "move care to the left." That is, management of a patient-initiated symptom may progress (from left to right) from a receptionist, to a nurse, then a physician extender, and finally to the physician. For frequently occurring problems, such as the common cold, physician visits are expensive and contribute little to patient welfare. "Moving care to the left" involves more patient education and self-treatment, with attendant cost savings and a reduction in inappropriate use of health care resources. However, for problems such as the common cold, the actual reduction in health care cost is relatively minor, since a physician visit alone is comparatively inexpensive.

The osteopathic emphasis on prevention and nutrition can promote an application of this concept to more complex disorders, such as the treatment of hypertension, diabetes, and coronary heart disease. For example, osteopathic physicians have long promoted the role of lifestyle changes in the management of these common problems by recommending regular exercise, proper diet, and weight loss. Such treatment may be effective in eliminating, reducing, or delaying the need for pharmacological management and is consistent with the early history of osteopathic medicine as a drug-free profession.

The problem of hypercholesterolemia is one for which osteopathic medicine may represent an inherently natural approach.[14] The widespread use of lipid-lowering medications or large-scale screening for hypercholesterolemia in the general population is not recommended. Rather, a targeted approach aimed at the identification and treatment of high-risk individuals does appear to be warranted. The best screening method is a visit to the primary care physician. With the exception of serum lipid levels, information needed to evaluate the patient's health status including family history, socioeconomic level, the presence of risk factors, and the patient's blood pressure reading can readily be obtained in the physician's office. Typically, persons with coronary artery disease have multiple risk factors, which are often interrelated, such as obesity, hypertension, elevated glucose levels, and dyslipidemia. The modification of these risk factors needs to be multifactorial, vigorous, and sustained.

The new cholesterol-lowering medications that inhibit HMG-CoA reductase, which are now known as the statins, have an unprecedented efficacy in lowering elevated serum cholesterol. However, the high cost of these lipid-lowering medications accounts for at least 70% of the estimated cost of all treatment strategies for patients with proven coronary heart disease. There are other methods for lowering serum cholesterol, including exercise, weight loss, and low-fat, high-fiber diets.

Are all cholesterol-lowering methods equal? Although clinical research data are not available, epidemiological studies would tend to support the idea that dietary intervention provides a different type of risk reduction, because a low-fat diet typically involves large amounts of fruits and vegetables, which are naturally rich in antioxidants.[23] Certainly, to prescribe a cholesterol-lowering drug without prescribing a low-fat diet and an exercise program makes no more sense than placing an obese diabetic patient on oral hypoglycemic agents without first intervening with diet and exercise. Recalling our heritage as a drugless healing profession, many proponents of a distinctive role for osteopathic medicine would suggest that drugs be used only after a vigorous effort has been made to lower cholesterol through lifestyle changes.

Too often, health care reform puts the primary care physician in the role of gatekeeper, and that individual is seen as blocking care, rather than providing appropriate care. In large part, this is an understandable reaction to occasionally unnecessary expenses that have occurred with a specialty referral. However, the implementation of the osteopathic precept of a rational treatment based on viewing the patient as a whole, structure/function relationships in the body, and the intrinsic self-regulatory features of the body can provide a framework for understanding the gatekeeper role of a primary care physician as one that is beneficial both to the patient and to the cost-containment component of health care reform.

A significant component of health care expense involves hospitalized patients. Here, managed care concentrates on attempts to divert the hospital visit, to manage emergency department admissions, to manage scheduled admissions, and to manage the hospital length of stay, all with the goal of reducing health care costs. The osteopathic specialist can play a major role in the development of policies that will express the osteopathic philosophy and, therefore, enhance the quality of patient care. For example, care paths have been developed to manage patient care of a variety of common conditions, such as acute myocardial infarction, unstable angina, hip replacement, and so forth. The initial goal of such programs was to reduce the length of stay in the hospital, and most major institutions continue to judge the value of such care plans in terms of hospital length of stay.

The osteopathic approach to such care plans would be to institute a care plan in order to enhance the quality of patient care, to improve the education of patients and family members, and to provide a foundation for the establishment of appropriate post–hospital care. The orientation of discharge planning should be directed towards selecting the proper care environment and providing medical resources to enhance the patient's ability to recover from the illness and to minimize the chance of a subsequent return to the hospital, especially because of lack of adherence to medication directions or to lifestyle changes. In some osteopathic hospitals, these care plans have been used to standardize the incorporation of services of osteopathic manipulative medicine into the hospital course.

A host of individuals are contending for control of the hospitalized patient, many motivated by financial concerns (hospital administrators, physicians, nurses, third party insurance carriers, the federal government) and an equally large group is involved in patient care (physicians, nurses, physical therapists, dietitians, social workers, discharge planners, etc.). The osteopathic philosophy represents an important perspective that the specialist can apply in the development of continuum care paths.

CHALLENGES

The reform of medicine will never be complete. Each year, new forces emerge that tend to erode the doctor-patient relationship and jeopardize the ability of the patient to be an active participant in a holistic care model. For the osteopathic profession, there are several challenges.

The first challenge that faces osteopathic specialty care is that of developing and maintaining distinctiveness in the training program. In a health care environment where financial concern is dominant over philosophy, more and more osteopathic hospitals have been closed or purchased by larger allopathic institutions. Where osteopathic hospitals continue to exist, frequently the education programs are combined with affiliated MD teaching institutions. Osteopathic postgraduate training programs need to develop strategies for comprehensive training programs that will integrate the osteopathic philosophy throughout the training program.

Promoting research in osteopathic medicine is another challenge. Osteopathic specialists have a key role to play in the promotion of research. For decades there has been constant pressure to develop research protocols to assess the efficacy of osteopathic manipulative treatment and other forms of osteopathic practice. In each research trial on the application of manipulative treatment, the specialist in manipulative medicine should work collaboratively with a specialist in the corresponding field of study. For example, a project on the efficacy of OMT in the treatment of asthma would involve a collaborative relationship between pulmonologists and OMT specialists, and a project on postoperative management of surgical patients would link surgeons with manipulative specialists.

The realization of the osteopathic concept becoming an integral part of health care is yet another challenge. Attempts to implement the osteopathic concept will meet persistent pressure from forces whose primary aim is to reduce health care costs. A lesser force in opposition will be dedicated to improving quality and cost effectiveness. These two goals are not incompatible, but before they can be achieved, answers must be found to important questions concerning the most efficacious means to treat common clinical disorders such as back pain, hypercholesterolemia, coronary heart disease, and diabetes. Third party insurance carriers and the federal government have considerable skepticism regarding the value of preventive care. Further, the osteopathic physician needs to find an appropriate balance in the use of lifestyle modification, pharmacological agents, and surgery for treatment of disease. The most "osteopathic" approach may not be that which is completely drug free or based on manipulative management, but rather that which is most acceptable and valuable for individual patients in their own specific clinical circumstances.

The greatest challenge to the osteopathic profession is that of establishing the context for health care reform. Presently, the initiative to lead this discussion is in the hands of politicians, the federal government (Health Care Financing Administration [HCFA]), third party insurance carriers, and the political structures within the American Medical Association and the American Osteopathic Association. The discussion of health care reform centers on the cost of care and only occasionally touches on the fundamental issues of concern to society, such as access to care and the plight of uninsured and underinsured persons. Simple and logical approaches to the reduction of costs, such as a single payer system, are rarely considered.

However, health care reform, as proposed by Irvin M. Korr, PhD, involves a much more fundamental issue than cost. Osteopathic medicine was established as an improvement on the present system. Korr points out that the central theme of the allopathic school of medicine, symbolized by Asclepius, is the concern for the afflictions to which man is heir and susceptible.[10] According to this system, diseases are viewed and treated as "autonomous entities." Whereas individuals differ in their susceptibility, resistance, and response to the various diseases, each of the diseases is nevertheless an entity with a natural history, subject only to minor modifications by the "host." In contrast, the osteopathic system of medicine, symbolized by Hygeia, is not the natural history of diseases, but of people.

From this viewpoint, disease and diseases are not merely the superimposed "effects" of adventitious "causes." They are not epiphenomena of pathological molecular and biological processes that intrude upon "life." They are life, life under unfavorable circumstances: those of disparity between the capacities, resources, and responses of the individual, on the one hand, and the demands and the circumstances of his life, on the other.[10] The patient's true illness, then, is not the disease, the particular aberration of organ, cell, or process. His illness is in his total being; it involves and reflects all the factors that make him a unique individual. The dominant forces of allopathic medicine, of the media, the popular press, and other forces in American society all enforce the viewpoint of the school of Asclepius. The promotion of the view of philosophy symbolized by Hygeia represents the predominant challenge to the osteopathic profession in its reform of medicine.

CONCLUSION

Osteopathic specialists have the potential to make manifold contributions to the process of the reformation of medicine in the United States. The primary role of the specialist is to assist in the growth of the osteopathic profession through clinical service (patient care). To this end, specialists integrate the tenets of osteopathic medicine in their practice and provide a perspective for the primary care physician that enhances comprehensive care. Osteopathic specialists can be helpful in determining in which cases osteopathic philosophy can be implemented with osteopathic manipulative therapy, recognizing that the exponential growth of diagnostic and therapeutic modalities has provided a sharper focus that more clearly defines the effectiveness of OMT. In addition, the osteopathic specialist has the opportunity to provide input on a modern interpretation of osteopathic tenets, to promote research within the osteopathic profession, and to provide leadership in terms of expanding osteopathic concepts. The greatest challenge to the osteopathic profession is shared equally by the specialist and the primary care physician, that is, to attempt to place on the agenda of health care reform the issue of true health care, one based on the natural history of people and how their bodies respond under unfavorable circumstances. This involves orientation to the patient and recognition that illness is in the total being, a viewpoint that runs contrary to the dominant forces of allopathic medicine, the popular press, and the health care "industry."

The author is grateful to Irvin M. Korr, PhD, for his thoughtful review of this manuscript.

References

1. Beal MC: Palpatory testing for somatic dysfunction in patients with cardiovascular disease, *JAOA* 82:822-831, 1983.
2. Chahan A, Mullins PA, Thuraisingham SI, et al: Effect of transcutaneous electrical nerve stimulation on coronary blood flow, *Circulation* 89:694-702, 1994.
3. Cox JM, Gorbis S, Dick L, et al: Palpable musculoskeletal findings in coronary artery disease. Results of a double blind study, *JAOA* 82:831-836, 1983.
4. Crea F, Gaspardone A, Kaski JC, et al: Relation between stimulation site of cardiac afferent nerves by adenosine and distribution of cardiac pain: results of the study in patients with stable angina, *J Am Col Cardio* 20:1498-1502, 1992.
5. Elkiss ML, Rentz LE: Neurology. In Ward RC, editor: *Foundations for osteopathic medicine*, Baltimore, 1997, Williams & Wilkins.
6. Emmanuelsson H, Mannheimer C, Waagstein F, et al: Catecholemine metabolism during pacing-induced angina pectoris and the effect of transcutaneous electrical nerve stimulation, *Am Heart J* 114:1360-1366, 1987.
7. Hallgren RC, Greenman PE, Rechtien JJ: Atrophy of suboccipital muscles in patients with chronic pain: a pilot study, *JAOA* 94:1032-1038, 1994.
8. Healy B: Endothelial cell dysfunction: an emerging endocrinopathy linked to coronary disease, *J Am Col Cardio* 16:357-358, 1990.
9. Kappler RE: Exercises and recovery. In Ward RC, editor: *Foundations for osteopathic medicine*, Baltimore, 1997, Williams & Wilkins.
10. Korr IM: The function of the osteopathic profession: a matter for decision. In *The collected papers of Irvin M. Korr*, Colorado Springs, Colo, 1979, American Academy of Osteopathy.
11. Mannheimer C, Carlsson CA, Emmanuelsson H, et al: The effects of transcutaneous electrical nerve stimulation in patients with severe angina pectoris, *Circulation* 71:308-316, 1985.
12. Nicholas AS, DeBias DA, Ehrenfeuchter W, et al: A somatic component to myocardial infarction, *Br Med J* 291:13-17, 1985.
13. Pasceri V, Cianflone D, Finocchiaro ML, et al: Relation between myocardial infarction site and pain location in Q-wave acute myocardial infarction, *Am J Cardio* 757:224-227, 1995.
14. Rogers FJ: Osteopathic medicine: an inherently natural approach to cholesterol reduction, (Editorial) *JAOA* 96:28-30, 1996.
15. Rosero HO, Greene CH, DeBias DA: A correlation of palpatory observations with the anatomical locus of acute myocardial infarction, *JAOA* 87:119, 1987.
16. Ross SP: General surgery. In Ward RC, editor: *Foundations for osteopathic medicine*, Baltimore, 1997, Williams & Wilkins.
17. Scott RA: Orthopaedics. In Ward RC, editor: *Foundations for osteopathic medicine*, Baltimore, 1997, Williams & Wilkins.
18. Shaw HH, Shaw MB: Ears, nose, and throat. In Ward RC, editor: *Foundations for osteopathic medicine*, Baltimore, 1997, Williams & Wilkins.

19. Special Committee on Osteopathic Principles and Osteopathic Technic, Kirksville College of Osteopathy and Surgery: An interpretation of the osteopathic concept, *J Osteopathy* 60:7-10, 1953.
20. Sucher BM: Myofascial manipulative release of carpal tunnel syndrome: documentation with magnetic resonance imaging, *JAOA* 93:127-128, 1993.
21. Sucher BM: Palpatory diagnosis in manipulative management of carpal tunnel syndrome, *JAOA* 94:647-663, 1994.
22. Tettambel MA: Obstetrics. In Ward RC, editor: *Foundations for osteopathic medicine,* Baltimore, 1997, Williams & Wilkins.
23. Verschuren MM, Jacobs DR, Bloemberg BPM, et al: Serum total cholesterol and long-term coronary heart disease mortality in different countries: twenty-five year follow-up of the seven country study, *JAMA* 274:131-136, 1995.
24. Vogel RA: Risk factor intervention in coronary artery disease: clinical strategies, *Coron Artery Dis* 6:466-471, 1995.
25. Ward RC, editor: *Foundations for osteopathic medicine,* Baltimore, 1997, Williams & Wilkins.

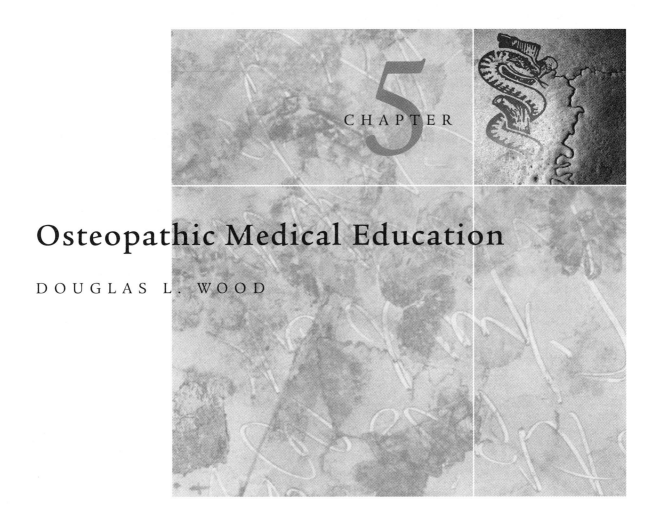

Osteopathic Medical Education

D O U G L A S   L .   W O O D

The past did not occur in an inevitable or predictable fashion; neither will the future. However, the past bears powerfully on the present in American medicine.[4]

KENNETH M. LUDMERER

HISTORY

The history of osteopathic medical education, like that of osteopathic medicine, is laced with richness, intrigue, successes, and failures. After having attached the name *osteopathy* to his new philosophy and practice of medicine, Dr. Andrew Taylor Still decided it must be taught to others and, thus, established the American School of Osteopathy in Kirksville, Mo in 1892. The first class of students consisted of 15 men and 3 women. The inclusion of women is unique in that very few females were admitted to medical schools in the late 1800s. Dr. Still was known to be an ardent liberal; he also opened the school to African Americans. The education of the first groups of students stood in stark contrast to current medical education. The mornings were dedicated to the study of anatomy without cadavers, and afternoon sessions consisted of working in the infirmary and observing Still put into practice his beliefs about the human body.[5] The "clinical education" of Still's students was enhanced in that patients usually agreed to stay in Kirksville for at least a month thereby allowing students an opportunity to observe the progress of patients over an extended period of time. Within a few years, the school in Kirksville had grown to over 700 students, and a number of new schools were being established elsewhere by Still's graduates.

By the early 1900s, a number of operating osteopathic medical schools closed. The rapid rise and fall in the fortunes of those schools that did not survive was brought on by two factors: (1) insufficient enrollment caused by too many schools for the number of prospective students and (2) a 1903 requirement that all colleges of osteopathic medicine start a 3-year, 27-month compulsory curriculum by September 1904. The requirement for the lengthened course of study came about as a result of an on-site survey conducted by the Associated Colleges of Osteopathy (ACO), which was established in 1898. The ACO was formed to develop a set of common educational standards to which the schools were expected to comply—admissions process, length and breadth of course work, curricular offerings, and clinical instruction.[2]

On a much larger scale than the ACO survey, the tour of the nation's medical schools, both MD and DO granting, by Abraham Flexner resulted in his well known and previously mentioned 1910 publication "Medical Education in the United States and Canada." Flexner noted numerous problems with osteopathic medical education and declared that not one "of the eight osteopathic medical schools is in a position to give such training as osteopathy demands." Flexner recognized that the MD and the DO approaches were different, yet he justified touring osteopathic medical schools by declaring, "Whatever his notions on the subject of treatment, the osteopath needs to be trained to recognize disease and to differentiate one disease from another quite as carefully as any other medical practitioner. . . Whether they use drugs or not does not affect this fundamental question. . . All physicians summoned to see the sick are confronted with precisely the same crisis: a body out of order. No matter what remedial measures they incline—medical, surgical, manipulative—they must ascertain what is the trouble. There is only one way to do that. The osteopaths admit it when they teach physiology, pathology, chemistry, microscopy."[1]

Although many within the osteopathic profession were deeply angered by the report, one group was not, the American Osteopathic Association (AOA) Committee on Education. It basically agreed with Flexner that the quality of osteopathic medical education was hampered by low entrance requirements, poor basic science laboratories, insufficient clinical facilities, and inadequate faculty. Three years after the report, the AOA Committee on Education developed a standard curriculum, and in 1915 a 4-year educational program was required of all AOA-endorsed osteopathic medical schools.[2] Other reforms suggested by Flexner have been addressed and implemented over time by osteopathic medical education.

The greatest strides in reform of the standards for osteopathic medical education did not occur until the latter half of the twentieth century. In the late 1930s and early 1940s, the schools began imposing an entrance standard requiring one year, and in some instances two years, of college before being considered. This requirement was gradually increased to the point that by 1960 nearly 71% of all new matriculants were entering with a bachelors or advanced degree and by 1998 that number was 99%.

The basic science curriculum was enriched by a higher percentage of time being spent in the laboratory and the hiring of full-time faculty with masters and doctorate degrees. The clinical side of the curriculum experienced an even greater transformation. The amount of bedside and outpatient experience per student rose from an average of 826 hours in 1935-1936 to 2214 hours in 1958-1959.[2]

The 1960s brought a growing consensus that the nation would soon experience a shortage of physicians since the number of medical school graduates was not keeping pace with the postwar population growth. This perception of a shortfall of physicians prompted a resurgence in the establishment of new osteopathic medical schools. While only five schools had survived the first 50 years of the osteopathic movement, 14 new colleges were established in its second 50 years. Within this span of 100 years, osteopathic colleges have educated 44,000 physicians.

OSTEOPATHIC UNDERGRADUATE MEDICAL EDUCATION

Several of the currently existing osteopathic medical schools stressed the continuum of medical education, which includes undergraduate medical education, graduate medical education, and continuing medical education. The American Association of Colleges of Osteopathic Medicine endorsed this continuum through the Osteopathic Postdoctoral Training Institution (OPTI) concept, and all schools now are working toward this end. Thus, once undertaken, medical education truly is a life-long venture.

Considerable evolution has taken place in osteopathic undergraduate medical education since the days of Still's one-room school, not only relating to the basic structure of osteopathic medical schools but also relating to the curricular models that are used. Relative to structure, reference has been made previously to the relationship between osteopathic medical schools and colleges and universities. The trend toward relatively tight bonding between the osteopathic medical schools and a university was started with the establishment of a medical school at Michigan State University. Of the 19 current colleges of osteopathic medicine, 11 are either part of a university or are part of a state system, such as the West Virginia School of Osteopathic Medicine or the University of Medicine and Dentistry of New Jersey–School of Osteopathic Medicine, which is one of three osteopathic colleges in state-supported research-intense universities. Although the physical structure of the medical school does not directly impact its function, there is some relationship (albeit decreasing with the increasing use of technology) between the two. A healthy diversity is found among osteopathic medical schools relative to their structure. Beyond the physical structure, several other components are necessary in order to "conduct" osteopathic undergraduate medical education. Some of these elements are curricular models, faculty, the student body, and clinical rotation sites.

In most U.S. medical schools, one can see varying degrees of definition between the preclinical and the clinical portions of the curriculum. The "standard" curriculum consists of 2 years spent in the preclinical phase and 2 years in the clinical phase. This is a model that was based on a Germanic tradition and thereafter transported to this country in what is known as the "2 + 2" curricular model. This particular model, in its pure form, is found in very few U.S. medical schools and no osteopathic medical school. The pure form of the model demands a clear demarcation between the basic science courses taken in medical school and the clinical portions of the curriculum. In today's increasingly integrated medical world the pure 2 + 2 model seems less and less appropriate. Despite what might seem to be shortcomings, a modified version of this model is still used in a moderate number of both allopathic and osteopathic medical schools. As the boundaries between the various basic science disciplines become increasingly blurred, this model will most likely be less and less appropriate.

The other two curricular models found in osteopathic medical education are the problem-based model and the organ systems curriculum. In allopathic medical education, the problem-based model has been gaining increasing prominence, albeit in a modified form when compared to what might be called a pure problem-based model. In the pure model, students during the first few months of medical school are provided with an introduction to the basic sciences and thereafter are divided into groups of 6 to 10 students who work together to solve medical problems that are presented to them. Guidance is provided by a faculty mentor. When approaching the problem, the group of students must consider both the basic science (anatomical, physiological, biochemical, and pharmacological components, to name a few) and clinical aspects of the problem. Via the use of the presented problems, students are expected to master basic science and clinical concepts in the context of the problem. Since one of the fundamental functions of the physician is problem solving, this model has much appeal to many who work in the area of undergraduate medical education. Despite its increasing use in the allopathic medical education environment, there still are drawbacks to employing the pure problem-based model. One of the major issues is that this model does not seem suited to all medical students and, as a matter of fact, may be well suited to only about 25% of medical students. It is also very faculty intensive, which is problematic in an era when faculty practice–generated monies, which are used for curricular support, are decreasing primarily because of the impact of the management of care. In osteopathic medical education, the pure problem-based model is offered as a special tract only at the University of Medicine and Dentistry of New Jersey–School of Osteopathic Medicine. The use of medical problems as a vehicle for the study of many aspects of health care is, however, gaining increasing favor in osteopathic medical schools.

Currently, the most widely used curricular model in osteopathic medical education is the organ systems model. This model was developed in the 1950s at what is presently known as the Case Western Reserve School of Medicine. The 1950s was a time of unrest and dissatisfaction with medical education and a time when medical education was looking for improved ways to educate medical students. The educators at Case Western conceived of a curricular model whereby more integration of the basic and clinical sciences could be accomplished. The model is usually integrated after the students have a fairly firm grounding in the basic sciences. Thereafter, the various body systems are studied, usually beginning with a review of the anatomy, physiology, biochemistry, and so forth of that particular system and then progressing forward to a study of the various diseases affecting that body system. Many schools that use this model teach the clinical aspects of each system using a problem-solving format.

The systems model seems especially well suited to osteopathic medical education. It allows an integrated approach as was stressed initially by Dr. Still when he spoke of the body functioning as a unit—thus all aspects of integration of a single body system can be seen by the student in one medical school course. Most osteopathic medical schools, through the use of problem-solving exercises, then allow the students to understand how all of the various body systems combine to create the integrated whole that is the human body.

In osteopathic as well as allopathic medical education, it is very difficult to find a medical school with a pure medical education model. Although occasional surveys ask medical schools to define the model used, in reality impure versions of the above mentioned models are employed in most U.S. medical schools. With the continual changes in health care, it will be necessary for medical education to continually evolve. Another factor to consider in any curricular design or model is the fact that all medical schools must adhere to standards required for the granting of the professional degree. At the same time, however, the curriculum must embody the unique characteristics that make each college of osteopathic medicine distinctive.

The clinical aspects of the osteopathic undergraduate medical school curriculum have some degree of uniformity across the schools. One aspect that is found in all of the schools is early exposure to patients, be they real or simulated (standardized). In most osteopathic medical schools, students are allowed to interact with patients during year one of their medical education. This is initially as an observer and subsequently with enhanced degrees of patient contact under close supervision. One part of early clinical exposure that is being increasingly used in osteopathic medical schools is the simulated (standardized) patient. These "patients" are individuals who are trained to simulate various disease states. Most experienced physicians are amazed at the skill of these "patients" as they mimic real patients. The simulated patient is of considerable advantage in examination situations in that they have been trained to present the same history and same physical examination findings across many students. These "patients" also can be trained to provide excellent feedback to students concerning student performance on both history taking and the physical examination.

It is obviously essential that medical students are exposed to real patients to an increasing degree as they progress along in their medical education. One unique aspect of osteopathic medical education has been patient exposure in community settings. Most osteopathic medical schools are not associated with large tertiary care medical centers but rather with community hospitals, clinics, and individual physician offices. Therefore, the majority of the clinical exposure of the osteopathic medical student takes place in these community-based facilities. Osteopathic medical students spend the majority of their time in the third and fourth years of medical school in clinical rotations, on such services as family medicine, internal medicine, pediatrics, surgery, and obstetrics/gynecology to name few. They also are allowed time on a variety of clinical electives. The continued emphasis on these rotations is to graduate a well rounded generalist rather than a student who has been oriented to a specific subspecialty during most of his/her clinical rotations. One may ask if it is not more appropriate for medical students to spend the majority of their time in large medical centers seeing very complex disorders as opposed to community settings. The answer to that from an osteopathic medical education perspective is "definitely not." Medical students must be exposed to the types of patients they will be seeing on a regular basis, and such exposure takes place in community settings and not in tertiary health are centers. This is not to say that medical students should not be exposed to patients with complicated conditions, but rather that these types of patients should not be their primary clinical exposure.

Another unique feature of osteopathic clinical education is that increasingly it is being conducted in the ambulatory environment. This is entirely appropriate in that there has been a significant movement of the practice of health care from the in-patient to the ambulatory setting over the past 20 to 25 years. It is currently felt that about 90% of all health care is delivered in the ambulatory arena. Does it not therefore seem logical to place medical students in the ambulatory environment for a significant part of their clinical exposure? There are physicians who argue against this approach stating that if medical students and, therefore, future practitioners can care for complex patients in in-patient settings they can care for just about any patient. This simply is not true for the types of patients and patient presentations seen in the ambulatory arena are often much different than those seen in hospitals. It is important that medical students to be exposed to both environments.

Throughout the curriculum, the osteopathic medical student is exposed to osteopathic principles and practice. They are taught the basic philosophy and principles upon which the profession is based and the clinical application of these principles. Much time is spent teaching the osteopathic medical students both palpatory diagnosis and osteopathic manipulative treatment techniques. Indications and contraindications for the use of these modalities are continually stressed to the end that they are used appropriately by the student and then in the practice life of these future osteopathic physicians.

Another component of the osteopathic medical school is the faculty. There are some differences between faculty in an osteopathic medical school and faculty found in an allopathic medical school. The faculty teaching in the basic science areas are generally quite similar, although there is some difference in their research interests, with an increasing number of basic scientists in osteopathic medical schools demonstrating research curiosity in the area of manual medicine (palpatory diagnosis and osteopathic manipulative treatment). In such topical areas as anatomy, there is a unique approach in that functional anatomy is stressed in osteopathic medical schools to a much greater extent than in allopathic medical schools.

There is a significant involvement of volunteer faculty in the teaching of the clinical aspects of medicine in osteopathic medical education. Although osteopathic medical schools have sufficient paid DO and MD faculty, there still is a cultural value placed on osteopathic physicians in private practice contributing actively to the clinical teaching. This donation of time and effort is felt by most physicians to be their contribution to the continuation of the profession and, of course, their opportunity to reap the benefits of teaching. Presently, osteopathic physician medical school faculty members are somewhat less involved in clinical research than are their allopathic counterparts, but a shift in this situation is taking place.

The last previously mentioned component of the osteopathic medical school is the student. Is there a difference in the osteopathic as opposed to the allopathic medical school student body? The answer here is "yes." Generally, osteopathic medical students are older than MD medical students, and many more of them are working on second careers. The latter partially accounts for the slightly lower medical college admission test (MCAT) scores of some students since more time separates their completion of college premed courses and their taking the MCAT's. Osteopathic medical students are also more likely to be married and also more likely to be a single parent. In addition, the osteopathic students are more likely to come from rural backgrounds, to have attended state or community colleges, and to come from less affluent families, which accounts for their higher debt on graduation, since many had to start borrowing money in college.

Accreditation of osteopathic medical schools is via the Bureau of Professional Education of the American Osteopathic Association. The Bureau has been approved by the United States Department of Education to be the accrediting body for osteopathic medical schools. To be accredited, an osteopathic medical school must demonstrate that it meets rigid standards and that it continues to meet these standards throughout its period of accreditation. The maximum period of accreditation of an osteopathic medical school is 7 years.

OSTEOPATHIC GRADUATE MEDICAL EDUCATION

Graduate medical education is the postgraduate training period an osteopathic physician must complete before practice.

In the early 1900s, the American Medical Association (AMA) sought to bar osteopathic physicians from any type of interaction within hospitals.[2] In the 1920s, the AMA facilitated legislation in several states that made medical school graduates eligible to take licensing examinations only after training in at least a 1-year graduate medical education program (internship). Since osteopathic medical students were denied access to allopathic hospitals, few internships were available to them. Because of this, osteopathic physicians had no choice but to build their own osteopathic hospitals to accommodate osteopathic medical school graduates. At the same time, specialty training programs (residencies) began to develop in the hospital as well. It was not until the 1960s that the AMA began to revise its stand on osteopathic physician training in allopathic hospitals. Now, nearly 50 years later, over 60% of DOs train in dual osteopathic/allopathic or allopathic programs. This is an amazing turnaround considering the historical biases held by allopathic physicians against their osteopathic peers.

In the osteopathic medical profession, the first year of graduate medical education training continues to be called the internship. Two types of internships are available: the rotating internship and the newer specialty internship. In the rotating internship program, the student is required to spend 4 weeks on a family practice service, 12 weeks on an internal medicine rotation, 12 weeks on surgery, 4 weeks on obstetrics/gynecology, 4 weeks on pediatrics, and 16 weeks of additional elective training. The emphasis on all of these rotations is an increasing level of education in the ambulatory environment. Even surgical rotations, which at one time were strictly conducted within hospitals, are now partially carried out in ambulatory surgical facilities.

Specialty internships are found in the areas of emergency medicine, family medicine, pediatrics, internal medicine, obstetrics/gynecology, psychiatry, and otolaryngology/facial plastic surgery. The internal medicine, obstetrics/gynecology, otolaryngology, and pediatric internships are specifically constructed so that the internship year can also be counted as the first year of residency training. Whereas each of the specialty internships has its own unique characteristics, all still contain elements of the rotating internship intermingled with a specialty training focus.

The residency is the training period following the internship year, wherein the student pursues further knowledge and skill in a specific area of medicine. The exception to this is in the areas of internal medicine, obstetrics/gynecology, otolaryngology, and pediatrics where the student is in a combined internship/residency program from the first graduate medical education year.

Currently, 76 separate specialty programs are approved by the American Osteopathic Association. In general, the osteopathic medical profession does not use the term *fellowship training* as is found in the allopathic profession, although many of the subspecialty programs are, in fact, fellowships. Specialty residencies include such programs as anesthesiology, emergency medicine, family practice, internal medicine, pediatrics, and general surgery, whereas subspecialty residency programs, for example, include cardiology, pulmonary, intensive care, endocrinology, infectious diseases, and vascular surgery. The success of the residency experience is built upon the strong generalist foundation the student obtained during undergraduate medical school and the internship. The residency period is also one during which knowledge and skills in osteopathic philosophy, principles, and practice are further enhanced. The resident has a unique opportunity to further explore the various distinctive features that distinguish the DO from the MD. The training in areas of medical practice that are considered more art than science, such as physician/patient interaction, is also augmented during the residency. By this time, the resident has a much greater appreciation of the many aspects and complexities of medical practice and therefore can better understand the importance of careful observation of teacher role models and of practicing observed techniques.

The residency period is also one during which many osteopathic physicians have their first direct experience in medical research, be it at the basic science or clinical level. Most osteopathic residency programs have a research requirement that serves to amplify the "spirit of inquiry," which must be found in any excellent physician. The amount of research production found in osteopathic medicine continues to increase partly as a result of the students' exposure to research experienced during the residency period.

An innovation in osteopathic graduate medical education is the so-called Osteopathic Postdoctoral Training Institution (OPTI), which was **fully** implemented July 1, 1999. Fundamentally, the OPTI concept dictates that all osteopathic graduate medical education must be conducted as part of a consortium by the above mentioned date. The fundamental components of an OPTI are an accredited osteopathic medical school, osteopathic health care facilities, ambulatory clinics, and other sites that qualify for recognition. The residency programs will be part of the OPTI and conducted as a partnership between the osteopathic medical school or schools involved and the health care facility or facilities. The OPTI must have a governing board that will oversee the entire operation of the consortium. Ultimately, the formation of graduate medical education consortia will continually enhance the quality of osteopathic graduate medical education and also promote the continuum concept in osteopathic medical education. The OPTI concept is fundamentally a new method of accrediting graduate medical education programs that holds much promise for innovation in accreditation. For many physicians, the completion of their residency program brings to a conclusion their formal education period. Yet undergraduate/graduate medical education must be viewed as only a part of the life-long learning experience of the physician. After the residency period, some physicians obtain further training in a subspecialty area; however, all physicians must participate in continuing medical education (CME) in order to maintain a license to practice medicine. Considering the rapid advances in both the diagnostic and therapeutic areas of medicine, physicians must commit to a lifetime of learning in order to effectively serve their patients.

FUTURE DIRECTIONS

Over the past decade medical education has carried out only modest attempts to reform its educational curricula. With the transformation taking place in American health care, medical education must reexamine its role in serving society and restructure its education process to better respond to the relevant needs of patients and the way health care is organized and delivered. Although osteopathic medical education is already meeting some of the demands of the emerging health care system—production of more generalist physicians, competence to practice in community-based and ambulatory care settings, and a curriculum focus on disease prevention and health promotion—the osteopathic curriculum will need to change to educate students in the competencies necessary for effective practice in the twentieth century. In particular, the osteopathic curriculum must shift to include the nine competence areas outlined by Dr. Nicole Lurie: "health systems finance, economics, organization & delivery; evidence-based epidemiologically-based medicine, ethics, development of patient-provider relationships, leadership; promoting teamwork and organizational change, quality measurement and improvement, medical informatics, systems based care, and competencies relevant to primary care (not specific to managed care)."[3] Those nine competencies are fundamental for any physician who desires to practice efficient and effective medicine in an environment where care is managed. Osteopathic medical education and medical education in general must move forward to include the teaching of all of these competencies in their medical education offerings.

Another area of concern currently, and definitely of concern in the future, is the expansion of medical knowledge and how it can best be monitored. Since all of the available medical information on even one body system could not be learned, one of the skills that must be mastered along the path of medical education is the ability to access information. Today's technology offers medicine a tremendous advantage compared to what was available only 10 years ago. Thus, the medical practitioner must be skilled in the use of computers, searching databases, and other related technology to access data.

The practice of health care requires cooperation among several persons or entities; for medical education to be effective currently and in the future, the same level of cooperation is required. The various bodies within the osteopathic profession that are concerned with osteopathic medical education must continually enhance their level of cooperation and collaboration. Likewise, the American Association of Colleges of Osteopathic Medicine (AACOM) must continue to elevate its level of cooperation with the Association of American Medical Colleges (AAMC).

With the transformation that is occurring in the way health care is and will continue to be managed and to ensure that health care is delivered in a way that best serves the public, the future direction of osteopathic medicine should look to the same goals that have guided it through its 100 years of history to date: (1) promotion of generalism; (2) production of distinctive physicians who practice osteopathic principles and techniques; and (3) promotion of access to care through appropriate geographic distribution of clinicians. To continue to promote and meet these goals, osteopathic medical education must continue to maintain authority over the educational continuum to assure that the generalist output continues to rise. It must continually enhance both undergraduate and residency training in the holistic orientation of patient care and the use of manipulative treatment. Finally, it must continue to make a concerted effort to foster practice in rural, underserved areas.

References

1. Flexner A: *Medical education in the United States and Canada—a report to the Carnegie Foundation for the Advancement of Teaching*, Boston, 1919, Marymount Press.
2. Gevitz N: *The D.O.s—osteopathic medicine in America*, Baltimore, 1982, Johns Hopkins University Press.
3. Lurie N: Preparing Learners for Practice in a Managed Care Environment, U.S. Dept. on Health & Human Public Health Service, HRSA, BHPr, Council on Graduate Medical Education, Resource paper, Sept. 1997.
4. Ludmerer KM: *Time to heal*, 1999, Oxford: New York, Oxford University Press.
5. Walter GW: *The first school of osteopathic medicine*, Kirksville, Missouri, 1992, Thomas Jefferson University Press at Northeast University State University.

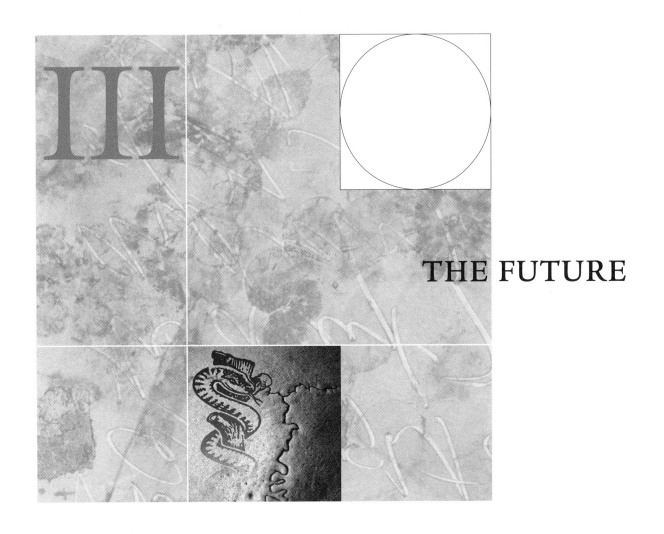

III

THE FUTURE

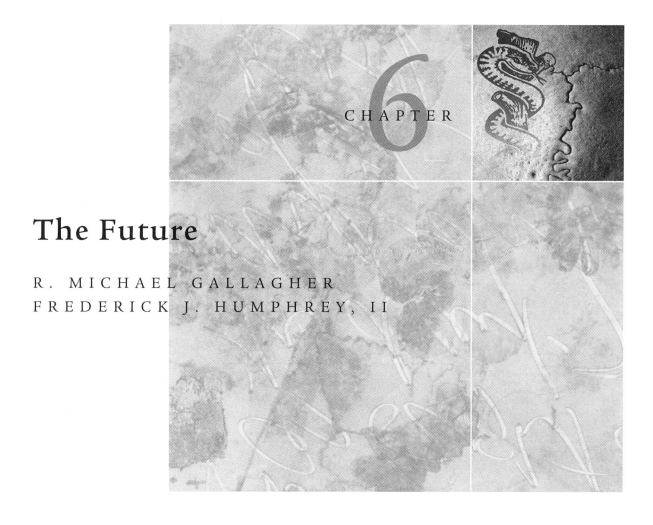

The Future

R. MICHAEL GALLAGHER
FREDERICK J. HUMPHREY, II

The best way to predict the future is to create it.

PETER DRUCKER*

he future, although perhaps impossible to predict, is something that we can help shape if we are prepared to be honest with ourselves regarding the realities that face us and are able to do what needs to be done. Osteopathic medical school administrators and heads of national and statewide osteopathic organizations have the responsibility to reflect on the osteopathic profession, where it has been and where it might be heading. Meanwhile, few osteopathic physicians on the frontlines of primary care take the time to get involved. All physicians are very busy, no doubt. But, all osteopathic practitioners need to be involved in addressing osteopathic medicine's future, on some level.

*Drucker P: *Management challenges for the 21st century,* New York, 1999, Harper/Collins.

Nothing less than the survival of the profession we have worked so arduously for is at stake.

If you ask any sizable group of osteopathic physicians at a given seminar, convention, or dinner meeting, "Where is the osteopathic profession heading?," members of the group often fall silent. Then, pose the more significant question: "Where should *we* be taking the osteopathic profession?" For without thought, discussion, and serious, open debate about our future, the real question might become, "*Is* there a future for osteopathic medicine?"

These are not questions for which there are easy answers. And these are not questions for which the answers will come overnight. Osteopathic physicians have had to work very hard to reach their present standing in medicine and in the community at large. Many osteopathic physicians are acutely aware of the history of their profession; many suffered professional prejudice. Far too many, once they achieved respected standing, have stopped there and become stuck: complacent and happy just to be practicing medicine, no longer feeling the need to fight for basic privileges.

For almost the entire history of the profession, until 1970, the educational and health care delivery systems were almost totally segregated, and there was very little public support. For the most part, DOs could only practice in osteopathic hospitals and referrals could only be made to other DOs. The question of who osteopathic physicians were was not an issue back then because the profession as a whole was defined by prejudice. It was clear who osteopathic physicians were. There was a sense that we had to take care of our own; no one was going to do it for us.

There was a strong volunteer spirit. Faculties were volunteer. The public began to notice that spirit and appreciate the personal touch osteopathic physicians shared with them and the attitude that each patient is an individual. They valued the willingness of osteopathic practitioners to try new modalities when traditional modalities failed.

Osteopathic physicians were at the vanguard. As progress was realized, osteopathic physicians focused on equal licensure, equal access to resources. Maintaining our identity was a nonissue since we were united in our struggle. Once the barriers were dropped, osteopathic physicians could practice in any hospital, and osteopathic medical students could apply for any residency program they would choose. We then began to recognize the importance of defining ourselves by our approach, our theory, our practice: the importance of holding onto our identity. That issue of identity now has moved to the forefront. It has brought up the question of exactly who are we and what do we do? In the struggle to prove we were equal to our allopathic brethren, had we lost our souls?

Today osteopathic medicine is growing in an unprecedented manner. But has our success been at the expense of an identity that is tied to a mission? Today osteopathic physicians practice in almost every conceivable environment and circumstance, in both osteopathic and traditionally allopathic institutions and settings. Whereas the number of allopathic institutions remains relatively constant, the number of osteopathic institutions continues to grow: 30 years ago there were 5 osteopathic schools in the United States; today, although the expansion is controversial, even within the profession, there are 19, with 3 new schools being founded in just the last 3 years. In 1989 there were 25,000 osteopathic physicians in the United States; at the turn of this twenty-first century, the American Osteopathic Association reports there are 44,000 DOs. On one level we have succeeded, yet still osteopathic physicians do not agree on exactly who we are.

It would appear that the osteopathic profession has at least three distinct choices for it's future: (1) By decision or by default (i.e., doing nothing), merge with the allopathic profession; (2) focus entirely on our historic strength and, in agreement with the allopathic profession, become medicine's primary care physicians; or (3) remain a distinct, but equal profession.

What would happen if the osteopathic profession merged with the much larger allopathic profession? Would this first option change the practice of medicine? Would we change? Would the public, and our patients, speak out?

Although osteopathic physicians and allopathic physicians work side by side in many institutions and settings, many allopathic physicians do not see their osteopathic brethren as distinctive in any way. Many allopathic physicians know only that osteopathic physicians have a different degree—different initials after their names—and they feel our differences are only historical.

Many, including Norman Gevitz, PhD, medical sociologist and historian at the Ohio University College of Osteopathic Medicine, feel that we are at risk of merging by default if either we or those in allopathic medicine feel there are no meaningful differences between us. If we are absorbed into the larger world of allopathic medicine, osteopathic medicine certainly would relinquish its most important role—that of a reform movement. Over the years, osteopathic medicine has developed very successful models for community-based medical education in primary care. Now, medicine is benefiting from our experience.

Some might argue that one centralized "brand" of medicine would simplify health care and medical education and potentially cut the skyrocketing costs of health care. Perhaps some officials in government do believe this to be the case, but at this point there is no way to know that is true. Others may feel that such an eventuality would even reflect the wishes of the majority of our members and afford us greater respect. They would also argue that allopathic medicine has embraced primary care medicine and that we are no longer distinctive. One might even take the opposite position: that having two major "styles" of medicine benefits both allopathic physicians and osteopathic physicians, medically and in terms of managing the cost of care. The fact is that osteopathic medicine has been managing costs all along, through its steadfast emphasis on primary care. Our system uses expensive specialists and special technology when it is necessary for diagnosis and treatment, but not as our primary response to patient care.

If allopathic medicine absorbed osteopathic medicine, how long would it take for the practice of osteopathic manipulative treatment to disappear? The entire hands-on approach probably would be left to chiropractors, since so few allopathic physicians understand or use OMT. Those patients who have come to rely on OMT for relief of back pain, neck pain, and headache would be without a modality that has helped them, in some cases, for many years. By relegating manipulative medicine to chiropractic, patients would not receive such treatment as part of an integrated medical approach that uses only medication and surgery as needed.

The second option of becoming medicine's primary care physicians is somewhat tempting, since it involves our niche as the generalist, experts in primary care. Also, this second option might negate the first one. It could protect osteopathic medicine and osteopathic medical education from being absorbed by allopathic medicine. It would ensure that osteopathic physicians would be able to practice according to their own precepts, while maintaining their own identity and distinctive nature. We would take advantage of our leadership in developing a training model that ensures that every graduate is well-versed in basic, primary care, which, in turn, has become a model for all of medical education. Managed care has seen to that.

Our history of emphasis on primary care positions us well to be leaders in the health care arena of tomorrow. Our knowledge and background in primary care would become more evident to the larger community, as this would become our official and publicized niche. The public, in far greater numbers, would look to osteopathic physicians for their primary care medical needs.

Becoming the purveyors of *only* primary care would enable osteopathic physicians to focus all of their attention on developing educational models in primary care, including serving as the medical educator to their patients. Osteopathic physicians, of course, would still teach their patients about the importance of preventive medicine, but they would do so to greater numbers of patients, who might realize for the first time what makes their doctor different, distinctive.

This option becomes even more tempting when you consider that as the number of osteopathic hospitals decline it becomes increasingly difficult to train osteopathic specialists in osteopathic hospitals. Focusing on primary care would allow osteopathic medicine to concentrate all of its resources in the primary care arena, leaving the specialty fields to allopathic medicine and defining and simplifying the role of the osteopathic clinical delivery system. A corollary of this argument is that our distinctiveness is limited to primary care medicine, and therefore, there is no justification for fighting to maintain our own specialty-training programs.

However, one needs to ask if losing our ability to train our own specialists would erode the way in which osteopathic physicians practice—limiting osteopathic practitioners to primary care when they might have a special talent in another area. That would cause them to leave the osteopathic profession for training and certification elsewhere. Is it not the breadth of knowledge of structure and function—the osteopathic physician's particular strength in general medicine—that lends a unique quality to the osteopathic specialist? This component of their medical practice emphasizes that what is being treated is the entire patient, not simply a body part or disease, even in the highly specific and technical world of the specialist. This approach adds great strength to the relationship between the specialist and the patient and between the patient and primary care physician—an important relationship that has significant implications for outcomes.

The third option, remain a different but equal profession, is most intriguing to us because it allows the osteopathic profession to live and work by its own tenets, while providing patients with an alternative, a choice. It also allows osteopathic medicine to continue in its role as a medical reformer, since osteopathic physicians have an impact on all medical specialties, not only on primary care.

A.T. Still started out to reform all of medicine. It can be argued that osteopathic medicine should exist as a separate entity until its precepts are incorporated into all medical school curriculums. **This reformation is not yet complete.** But simply deciding not to merge with allopathic medicine is not enough, since merger can occur regardless if we do not take strong actions. It is also not enough to say that historically we have been a reform movement. The latter is simply rhetoric unless we keep the reform movement alive by clarifying and promoting our medical philosophy. If osteopathic physicians want to remain free to practice osteopathic medicine, we need to know who we are and what we do. It is important that we have a better grasp of what makes osteopathic physicians different, distinct. It is about our identity. And osteopathic practitioners better be able to get it across to those outside the profession. This is paramount if we wish to see ourselves as reformers.

Unfortunately, perhaps because of a perceived lack of prestige relative to allopathic medicine, many osteopathic physicians seem unwilling to hold onto their roots. They are tired of being misunderstood by many in the public. Numerically, osteopathic physicians are a minority. And approximately 65% of our graduates enter American College of Graduate Medical Education (ACGME) programs for all or part of their training and are potentially lost to the osteopathic profession. Consider this: The American Academy of Family Physicians, which started admitting osteopathic physicians in 1993, now has more than 3300 DO members, many of them quite active. These are examples of precisely why the status quo will not work; why osteopathic medicine needs to move forward, if it wishes to be a separate and distinct profession.

Far too many osteopathic physicians take for granted who they are and what they do. "Osteopathic medicine is both a profession and a social movement," Ohio

University College of Osteopathic Medicine's Dr. Gevitz explained to the New York Times in a 1998 article about the osteopathic profession being on the rise after suffering years of scorn and derision. "It has to demonstrate that it can offer something distinctive, unique, and beneficial to the patient that allopathic graduates cannot offer. If osteopathic physicians become interchangeable with M.D.'s then there's no compelling reason for the profession to exist," emphasizes Dr. Gevitz, professor and chair, Department of Social Medicine.

Dr. Gevitz notes that for the osteopathic profession to promote its image—a distinct, recognizable identity—it must have a working definition: one that says who we are and what we do in clear, simple, brief, conversational English. It is the starting point from which those outside the profession can begin to ask questions about who osteopathic physicians are and what osteopathic physicians do; what makes us different.

In a July 1998 report by the American Osteopathic Association Task Force on Osteopathic Unity, chaired by Eugene Oliveri, DO, reporting to the AOA Board of Trustees, it was suggested that the AOA adopt, with modifications, the definition originally proposed by Dr. Gevitz:

> Osteopathic medicine is a complete and distinctive, primary care–centered approach to medical, surgical, obstetrical and other health services, founded on the importance of hands-on evaluation and treatment of the total person, and dedicated to the furtherance of health care for all people.[1]

What do you think? Which of the three options do you propose? If we opt to continue as a separate profession, working out exactly who and what osteopathic physicians are seems simple enough. But it is a daunting task as osteopathic medicine is met with a veritable plethora of opinions coming from every conceivable corner of the osteopathic profession. Through working out these kinds of problems and developing common goals, the osteopathic profession can flourish and reestablish its credentials as a reform movement, using the profession's special skills in primary care and OMT to take a leadership role in meeting the health needs of our society, taking the opportunity to be out front in the transition from hospital-based care to ambulatory care. The osteopathic medical schools will need to be ready to respond to the changing health care environment. Osteopathic medical students need to fully understand and be able to function with a high-level of competence in the ambulatory arena as the health care delivery system increasingly moves away from long-term hospital stays, and health maintenance organizations (HMOs) set the tone for the immediate future and, perhaps, beyond.

Individual osteopathic physicians need to further develop their greatest strengths: that as the purveyors of primary care and preventive medicine. Preventive medicine is somewhat of a double-edged sword. On one hand, everyone, it seems, is talking about the importance of preventive medicine. On the other hand, HMOs do not always view the essential nature of preventive care through the same lens as do osteopathic physicians. Osteopathic practitioners need to get the point across that it is not only better for the patient to be able to prevent disease and injury, but also better for society, economically and otherwise. In the area of primary care, the profession is right in step with the times. The allopathic system has had to refocus its ideas about its medical schools and graduates, changing from a model that focused on educating and training specialists and subspecialists to that of the primary care model, one which the osteopathic profession embraced long ago and never let go. As osteopathic physicians, we are in an excellent position to see through the changes in managed care, which favors a primary care physician overseeing patient care.

Osteopathic medicine will need to continue its emphasis on primary care. More than 50% of all practicing DOs are in primary care. Although only 5% of physicians in the United States are DOs, 10% of all physicians in primary care are DOs. This is a direct result of staying the course, staying true to osteopathic ideals and the osteopathic mission. When the allopathic system steered a course toward specialties and subspecialties, the osteopathic profession continued true to its mission, turning out some of the finest primary care physicians in the United States. Even osteopathic specialists carried the strength of their osteopathic training in primary care with them into other areas, making them more complete physicians, better able to see the complete picture, the complete patient. In short, we maintained our patient focus rather than adopting a disease focus. But we cannot assume that we will continue to produce the same percentage of primary care physicians without hard work on our part, since percentages have been dropping as more and more graduates enter ACGME programs.

The need for an agreed-upon definition brings us to another issue: promoting better visibility for the profession, which is critical no matter which option is chosen, but especially if we wish to maintain our status as a separate profession. So, mentioning primary care in any working definition of who we are makes sense. In its report, the AOA Task Force on Osteopathic Unity named two major objectives:

- Raise the visibility and accentuate the distinctiveness of osteopathic medicine to the public
- Revive the sense of distinctiveness within the osteopathic profession that recaptures the excitement and vitality of the movement begun more than 100 years ago by A.T. Still to reform medicine (A.T. Still attempted to present his idea to orthodox medicine. He founded his school only after being rejected by orthodox medicine.)

These objectives are of particular importance in light of surveys that show that up to half of respondents perceived no difference between osteopathic and allopathic medicine. Some illustrative examples:

- A 1981 survey, commissioned by the AOA, found a low level of awareness of osteopathic medicine among Ohio residents
- A 1996 survey at Michigan State University found that many osteopathic physicians spend a great deal of time explaining themselves to their patients

- A 1998 survey, commissioned by the Michigan Osteopathic Association, indicated that a fairly low percentage of respondents were aware of the distinctiveness and philosophy of osteopathic medicine

It is absolutely paramount that people know and understand who osteopathic physicians are and what osteopathic physicians do. This, of course, applies to the public (the patients), but it also applies to insurers and the government and to osteopathic medical students and even to young osteopathic physicians.

The need for greater visibility and a distinct identity places the osteopathic profession in the unique position of being able to do something about its image. Osteopathic physicians and others are in a position to have a great impact on the way in which the osteopathic profession is viewed by those on the outside. Sometimes, this means taking the time to explain osteopathic medicine. This can be time-consuming, but it also can be worth the time as outsiders begin to understand the message and pass along their new understanding and enlightened view to others.

As many osteopathic physicians begin to reopen their eyes to just what makes them different, it is very important to be open to the idea that every encounter is one in which the profession's message can be gotten across. Sometimes this can be done with great subtlety, other times it may call for a more straightforward approach, depending on the situation and the audience. But it does need to be done, and not just among practitioners, but also among students in osteopathic medical schools. This new understanding would increase the demand for the services of osteopathic physicians, since patients who are unfamiliar with the osteopathic profession or those who have been laboring under false ideas about the profession would then begin to appreciate the benefits of osteopathic medicine and seek a physician schooled in this philosophy. Even health care professionals outside of osteopathic medicine and government officials must be made aware of the distinctiveness of osteopathic medicine. Far too many of them, it seems, do not understand what osteopathic physicians do.

Greater visibility has many practical implications. For example, it could make it far easier for osteopathic physicians and institutions to obtain managed care contracts in this highly competitive marketplace in which today's winners could become tomorrow's losers. It is clear that the osteopathic profession's vision for the future is inextricably linked to how and what osteopathic medical students are taught. Perhaps former Surgeon General C. Everett Koop, MD, had osteopathic medicine in mind when he said: "When I say primary care, I mean the caring of patients. I don't know whether it was by teaching, by precept or by tradition, but osteopathic physicians have always understood that women and men are a

C. Everett Koop, MD, ScD: Former Surgeon General of the United States; Senior Scholar, The Koop Institute at Dartmouth, Hanover, New Hampshire; Chairman, National Museum of Health Medicine Foundation, Washington, DC.

trinity. They are souls, that they inhabit bodies, and they have a spirit. I think the people who really initiated whole person medicine and made it a formality in this country were osteopathic physicians. I think all of us should take our hats off to you about that."[2]

Osteopathic medical students must be well versed in the basics: in structure and function and in anatomy and physiology. And they must have a detailed understanding of hands-on techniques and of incorporating hands-on approaches along with other modalities. They must be able to marry a greater understanding of complex technology with a great compassion for their patients. Osteopathic medical instructors need to double their efforts to impart a strong foundation for osteopathic principles and practice (OPP) and OMT. Textbooks such as the *Foundations of Osteopathic Medicine,* can help in ensuring that all osteopathic medical students are well grounded in these basics and that they use a common language when discussing OPP, which must be a unifying theme in the curriculum.

An osteopathic medical education would not be balanced and grounded in the basics if it did not include study of how the osteopathic profession arrived at its current state. How can the doctors of tomorrow take the osteopathic profession to the next level if they are not fully aware of where it has been? We need to review our curriculum to learn if we need additional classroom instruction in the history of osteopathic medicine and the reform movement started by A.T. Still. We are sure that we all can agree that this would better prepare students for their careers, clarify the value of osteopathic medicine, and foster unity of purpose among the students and among medical educators.

It is true that the practice of modern medicine has become overcomplicated, filling physicians' time with patient care, keeping up with advances, practice management, and dealing with the ever-changing and ever-challenging world of managed care and more. It is no surprise, then, that the great majority of osteopathic physicians do not take the time to think about the profession's collective future. Perhaps many in the profession are too mired in individual, daily responsibilities and concerns to worry about the future of the profession: Somehow, it seems distant from what we do; we have lost our focus on the big picture. It is not really distant, though. The future is who we are and what we will become. There is no more important question facing the osteopathic profession, today. It is worth thinking about. It is worth your time. It is the future of the profession you have chosen. It is *your* future.

Many in osteopathic medicine know the history: How A.T. Still saw a medical establishment that was not filling many needs that needed to be filled. He saw a need for the pursuit of knowledge of the body as a composite and he pursued it. He saw the need for reform and he launched a tireless reformation. Certainly, Dr. Still's teachings were of medicine. But they also were of an approach to the future, a future that he opened up and one that osteopathic physicians further forged and evolved, until today, when osteopathic practitioners have become mainstream. How different it is to be battling the mainstream so arduously for so many years and then, finally, to join it—to, in many ways, link forces with allopathic physicians and institutions in matters that decades ago never would have been proposed.

Progress has been made. The osteopathic profession has earned respect. Osteopathic physicians are better off than they were decades ago. But in the process, the profession has lost sight of its mission and some of its identity: the sense of some of what makes osteopathic physicians different.

Reaching out with the message of the osteopathic profession can be accomplished with far less difficulty than one might surmise. Think about your education, training, and practice philosophy. Communicate your ideas and the ideals of the profession. Professional dialogue, whether physician-to-physician, physician to groups of physicians, or panel discussions, can go a long way toward bringing the profession from the individual mindset to the collective mindset, a place osteopathic physicians need to reach to ensure a future as a professional entity. This needs to be done on the local, state, regional, and national levels. For example, say you are at a panel discussion being presented for physicians and other medical professionals, government officials, or the public. Be sure people know that you are an osteopathic physician. Some osteopathic physicians might be surprised to learn how few osteopathic physicians refer to themselves as such.

Once osteopathic physicians are talking more about the future among themselves, the need will shift to reaching others. It is vital that osteopathic physicians get their message across in clear, simple terms to government officials, students in osteopathic medical schools, the media, the public, and to patients. In other words, the osteopathic profession should reach out to just about everyone. This "reaching" should be part of the profession's fabric, since how it is perceived will be, in large part, responsible for the profession's role in the future of medicine.

Only through reaching out and successfully getting the message across are osteopathic medical schools and institutions more likely to receive funding from philanthropists and from corporations that look to increase the scope of osteopathic education and research. Dr. Gevitz proposed a solution to what he terms "Osteopathic Invisibility Syndrome," in which each and every osteopathic physician contributes a small percentage of his or her gross annual income to a fund that would be used to promote the osteopathic profession. The AOA's Task Force on Unity also called for osteopathic physicians to make a financial contribution to the effort. Certainly, these suggestions or similar ones demonstrate the crossroads at which the entire osteopathic profession is standing; it illustrates the seriousness of the situation and makes us ask just how aggressive need we be?

If we wish to continue either as a primary care profession or a full profession, what is needed is nothing short of a revival among osteopathic physicians. What is necessary is a massive publicity campaign to start to make the world aware of who osteopathic physicians are and how they're different. Osteopathic medicine has been extremely successful, but in many ways it is still a secret. Many leaders in the osteopathic profession have applauded this "blue ribbon" committee to direct a major public education and promotional campaign and form a clear map for the road ahead. The osteopathic profession needs to develop a plan and then take it on the road.

Once everyone understands what is necessary, there needs to be a fund-raising effort that will enable the profession to turn its attention to the external environment. DOs need to reach the powers that be and need to reach the public. People need to know who osteopathic physicians are and what they do. This necessitates greater participation and membership in the AOA and other osteopathic medical organizations. We all have to ask ourselves if we have been as active as we should be.

Start with those who make the laws. By speaking with and writing to legislators, the profession becomes a voice that is heard. This point is paramount in maintaining our identity, as some government officials may work to consolidate state medical schools that now turn out either osteopathic or allopathic graduates. If these entities are not solidly convinced of the profession's worth and distinctive nature, they will attempt to meld osteopathic medical schools together with allopathic medical schools—in the name of saving money. This is one way in which a de facto merger can occur. There are an untold number of issues facing the osteopathic profession that could be directly or indirectly affected by elected officials. The more they hear from osteopathic physicians and those interested in osteopathic medicine, the more respect the profession will earn and the greater autonomy and equality the profession will enjoy.

Take the osteopathic profession's message to the streets. A voice unheard is a voice that receives no respect and no consideration. If you want the public to continue to view your profession as a wise and popular choice, and want that view to continue expanding, you need to reach the public, by speaking to service organizations and volunteer groups, by speaking at public lectures and question and answer sessions at hospitals and clinics, and by ensuring your voice is heard in myriad other public forums.

Take the osteopathic profession's message to the media, and let them reach the public and the decision makers. Try writing opinion articles to newspapers and magazines, and make yourselves available as medical experts; comment to the newspaper, radio and television reporters on every aspect of health care. Within this framework, osteopathic physicians will be able to impart not only critical medical information and advice, but also the very philosophy of the profession, down to its history of service in rural and urban underserved areas. A greater presence in these arenas is half the battle.

All of this discussion of the future of osteopathic medicine has great impact on the entire profession. But the real impact will be felt by today's students of osteopathic medicine. Mentors, teachers, regular physicians on the frontlines, and leaders in the profession need to take every opportunity to speak with students about the medical world they will inherit and about the importance of keeping their profession—and yours—alive. Now, more than ever, they need to know their history. They need to know where they have been if they are to know where they are going. The simple truth: They are the future of osteopathic medicine, and if they are not convinced that the profession is worth fighting for, it will die. Our time will soon be over. Only our students can ultimately ensure our future.

That brings us to one of the most important groups of all—the patients. Do you know why they chose an osteopathic physician to handle their health care? It is important to know. Some of them may have specific reasons; some of them may not. Some will understand the basic differences and similarities between osteopathic physicians and allopathic physicians, and some will not. It is important, in a very subtle way, to communicate your philosophy to your patients. Talk with them about approach, explain why you are handling a particular matter in a particular way.

We need to redouble our efforts in preventive medicine and in establishing and maintaining wellness. Remember your rigorous training in anatomy, the field that Dr. Still emphasized with such strength and conviction, the field on which he built his vision of osteopathic medicine. Tell your patients, when it is warranted, that you have highly specific training and experience in osteopathic manipulative therapy, which has been proven many times over to relieve musculoskeletal pain, headache, and more. Explain that your extensive training in primary care makes you particularly well-equipped in the areas of diagnostics and treatment, whether you are in general practice medicine or in a specialty. Work at being approachable, at being accessible. When patients feel they can put their complete trust in you, you will be paid back many-fold—and along the way, so will the entire osteopathic profession.

Osteopathic medicine's continued emphasis on primary care has stood the test of time. These days it is the subspecialist who feels the pressures being applied by managed care and by elected officials and bureaucrats. And this trend is projected to continue into the foreseeable future. This does not mean that the osteopathic profession should forsake the specialties or cease pushing for advancements toward a greater understanding of health and illness or advancements in developing new medical interventions and technology. Rather, osteopathic physicians should continue to integrate these ideas to better serve their patients, collectively and individually, and to set an example that continues to set the profession apart and reveals its practitioners as special.

The status quo was not good enough for Dr. Still—and it should not be good enough for osteopathic practitioners of today. A proactive approach, as discussed above, is critical. Merely attempting to hold on to what already has been accomplished will not be nearly good enough as pressures from outside the profession continue to mount. What is needed is osteopathic medical school students who cast an eye toward the future and osteopathic medical school administrators and instructors who provide a first-rate osteopathic medical education that is consistent, in its quality, from one osteopathic institution to the next.

The profession needs to reclaim its interest in osteopathic manipulative medicine. If you believe it will help in certain situations, use it. Do not let an entire modality remain in the closet. OMT is one of the profession's greatest assets, yet many osteopathic physicians, who could use this therapy, in combination with other medical modalities, choose to forego it. The results of a study published in a 1997 issue of the Journal of the American Osteopathic Association showed that far too few osteopathic physicians in family medicine treated half or more of their patients with OMT.[3]

Why are these techniques, even in combination with other modalities, now used far less than years ago? That is a question that is difficult to answer. Perhaps, many of these physicians fought for equality and acceptance for so long that they suppressed using a skill that they felt might only, once again, set them apart. Perhaps managed care, which places such strong emphasis on the amount of time spent with each patient, has brought pressure to bear? Or is it a lack of emphasis and a paucity of training in OMT, across all disciplines, in osteopathic medical schools? It is important to keep these skills alive and thriving beyond the classroom; they must be continued to be nurtured and depended upon in the clinical setting.

Training in OPP and OMT should not cease when an osteopathic medical student graduates from school. There is a strong need to continue training in these areas in postgraduate courses, and instructors should develop new and better ways of teaching these skills to osteopathic physicians, whether they are in osteopathic Graduate Medical Education (GME) programs or in allopathic GME programs. And according to the AOA's Task Force on Unity, "It is important to provide osteopathic physicians who have forgone an AOA-approved rotating internship with training in osteopathic medicine and a pathway to certification and membership in the AOA, and to continuing to provide physicians with opportunities to advance their knowledge in osteopathic principles and practice."[1]

As in all areas of medicine, osteopathic physicians must support research projects that will help the profession demonstrate which techniques are efficacious and which ones should be modified or abandoned. Publishing in this area, both in medical journals and in articles and books for the general public would go a long way toward demystifying OMT and in reestablishing osteopathic physicians as leaders in this area. This research is extremely important in terms of our serving as a reform movement since our goal is to change all of medical practice.

OMT is only one area, albeit a major one, in which osteopathic physicians must establish a research presence. The medical schools must lead the way, working with teachers and accomplished graduates to establish a basic and applied research base from which to launch a wide variety of projects that will have clinical implications. This is critical for our credibility with "internal publics" and for those outside the profession. This may be accomplished through the aggressive pursuit of grants from both the private and public sectors and by setting up a network of cooperation and shared information among the osteopathic medical schools.

Research brings distinction to the schools and to the researchers, and ultimately to the entire osteopathic "family." Publicity generated from successful research is yet another method of getting across the value of the osteopathic profession to the public and to government officials.

And what of the schools? It is not enough that year after year osteopathic medical schools continue turning out the highest percentages of physicians who will work in primary care. More needs to be done. Osteopathic medical educators need to step back and look carefully at our growth patterns. Quality in everything we do needs to be the highest priority. When we grow beyond our resources we endanger ourselves. For example, our growing reliance on allopathic GME programs makes us vulnerable by virtue of our inability to control our own destiny.

Osteopathic medical schools need to recruit more students who show a strong desire for and commitment to osteopathic principles. And the schools need to develop short-term, intermediate-term, and long-term approaches to improving osteopathic medical education.

No less an authority than George W. Northup, DO, FAAO, editor emeritus of the Journal of the American Osteopathic Association, called for students in osteopathic medical schools to be "well indoctrinated in the basic principles of the osteopathic medical profession," when he wrote his 12-part "Osteopathic Manifesto Series" for the JAOA, which was originally published beginning in February 1981 and reprinted after Dr. Northup's death in December 1996. "As our educational programs succeed, so does the profession," he wrote. "Osteopathic medical education is truly the light of the profession. It must never be allowed to dim. It must only grow brighter."

Meanwhile, more and more of the profession's hospital network and clinical delivery system is being eroded by the fast-changing patterns in health care policy and reimbursement. Because the osteopathic profession is smaller, it is more difficult to keep up. But, again, a smaller ship can make a faster turn than a larger one—and we must learn to project the changes that are coming and move proactively to maintain our viability and control over our own clinical systems.

The Osteopathic Postgraduate Training Institution (OPTI) should help in this regard. The OPTI program was established in part to ensure greater involvement of osteopathic medical schools to enhance the actual and perceived quality of osteopathic GME. By July 1999, all osteopathic residency training programs were required to be part of an OPTI, which includes an osteopathic medical school.

Any loss of control over our own clinical delivery system represents a threat to the osteopathic GME system as well. All of this makes competing for continued funding, in a fiscally tight environment, quite difficult. This is especially trying for osteopathic medical schools that receive state funding. In this environment, some elected officials could begin to question why they should continue to support osteopathic medical schools financially. This is yet another reason why it is paramount to get our message across to legislators—they hold the purse strings.

If we choose to remain a separate profession we need to remember that more than 60% of osteopathic medical school graduates attend American College of Graduate Medical Education training. In other words, many graduates from DO schools are receiving advanced medical training at MD institutions. Those who are "lost" to the osteopathic profession in this manner may become less inclined to stand up for the distinctiveness of their own profession. This translates to fewer soldiers in the war to remain equal, but separate. By continually teaching osteopathic medical students about their distinctiveness, many of them will be more inclined to choose osteopathic GME training. Expanding and enhancing this system also will make it a more attractive option for osteopathic medical school graduates, which, in turn, adds to the strength of the osteopathic profession.

Today much of what osteopathic physicians do depends far too much on the assistance of allopathic medicine and its institutions. For now, osteopathic medicine fits into their plans. But as the health care arena continues to evolve and resources are shifted or decreased, will osteopathic physicians still have access? At present, that is a question without an answer. Both now and in the future, the profession's greatest protection will come from its own systems, its own educational and training processes, and its own strength.

If we wish to remain separate, this is what is needed:

- A revival that centers around what makes osteopathic medicine distinctive as a profession
- Improved communication among all osteopathic physicians—especially between primary care physicians and specialists—to foster better understanding of one another and to better promote the profession's distinctiveness and identity
- A joining together for the common good of all osteopathic medical institutions, colleges, and clinical systems, be they large or be they small
- An understanding that anyone practicing osteopathic medicine or closely associated with an osteopathic physician, school, institution, and so forth has an obligation to promote and explain the osteopathic profession to those who might not understand it— since we all have something at stake

We need the help of everyone and every institution in the profession and all of those who care deeply about it to maintain the strides that have been made to this point and to move ahead and become even stronger. It is a necessity.

We are in this together. Join in.

References

1. Report by the AOA Task Force on Osteopathic Unity to the AOA Board of Trustees, July 7, 1998.
2. Video tape "A Walk Through History," commemorating the 100th Anniversary of the Philadelphia College of Osteopathic Medicine (PCOM), opening remarks by C. Everett Koop, MD, ScD, April 29, 1999.
3. Johnson SE et al: Variables influencing the use of osteopathic manipulative treatment in family practice. *Journal of the American Osteopathic Association*, 97:2, February 1997.

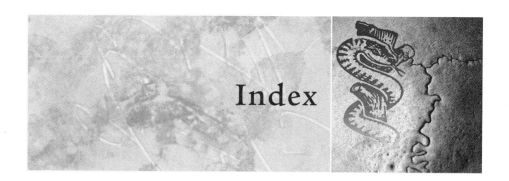

Index